BODY FIT

A Beginner's Guide to Fitness

BODY FIT

Greg Marshall

Familius LLC

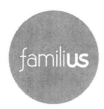

Published by Familius LLC, www.familius.com

Familius books are available at special discounts for bulk purchases for sales promotions, family or corporate use. Special editions, including personalized covers, excerpts of existing books, or books with corporate logos, can be created in large quantities for special needs. For more information, contact Premium Sales at 559-876-2170 or email specialmarkets@familius.com

Library of Congress Catalog-in-Publication Data
2013933807

pISBN: 978-1-938301-23-0
eISBN: 978-1-938301-24-7

Printed in the United States of America

Book design by Kurt Wahlner
Photography by Mike Young
Edited by Tabitha Thompson

10 9 8 7 6 5 4 3 2 1

First Edition

Contents

Introduction

Me and You

How I Got Here

I was initially attracted to the fitness industry because of the people in it and what the industry *really* represents—which is much more than six-pack abs and sexy body parts. Fitness can change your life forever by changing your mentality about yourself.

I originally got hooked when I was a kid, watching the amazing feats of the bodybuilders and fitness competitors I saw on television. It was like nothing I had ever seen. The competitors were so excited and energetic. And I couldn't help but feel the enthusiasm they had. It looked like they had a lot of fun and that they genuinely enjoyed being fit and healthy. From that point on I knew that I wanted to be as active and excited as they were.

I started out playing sports like baseball and absolutely loved how physical activity made me feel. I loved the competition against other people, but I enjoyed the competition with myself even more. Whether or not my team won was less relevant to me than whether my performance improved with each game. When I didn't do well,

I practiced and drilled until my performance was better. In a way, that's what fitness is: a constant effort to get better on any level, whether it is nutrition, resistance training, cardiovascular training, or even mental training. The goal is to push yourself to get better even on the days that you don't feel like pushing yourself.

As I began to excel in sports, the competitive, hungry side of me could not settle with being just "good." I wanted to meet my greatest physical potential. One day I read a fitness magazine with a professional athlete on the cover. The article inside explained how lifting weights and working out helped this athlete improve his sports performance. I must have read that fitness magazine from front to back dozens of times studying exactly what it was this athlete was doing to get better.

I used that article as a starting point to create my own daily workouts to see what results I would get and whether the work would translate into a better performance on the baseball field.

It worked! I quickly started to see great improvement of my abilities. There were just so many benefits that I was gaining from exercising and focusing on nutrition, resistance training, and cardio. The fitness industry stole my heart. I was in love.

But there's more to this story.

Working hard is never easy and I had some self-esteem issues to work through, as well. I want you to know that I understand where you're coming from and that I can help you work through it to get in great shape, no matter where you are starting.

Embrace Yourself, *Then* Better Yourself

I wasn't born with an athletic build. I was ridiculously smaller and skinnier than the rest of the guys my age. So even when I started doing really well in sports, I still felt inadequate because I wasn't as muscular or powerful as the others. Let's be honest, a male—especially an athletic male—wants to look powerful and unstoppable. Of course, the desire to feel successful is common to both genders in various parts of their lives. But in the world I was in, it was everything to me.

I really struggled because my body type didn't fit the athletic profile. And I was told there was nothing I could do to change it. I was told to just accept it. Being stubborn, though, I was determined to challenge that assumption.

In our society there are a lot of social pressures for men and women to meet a certain idealized body type. Any time we feel like we don't measure up to what we are "supposed" to be, it is really disheartening—especially when there doesn't seem like any way to better our situation. But there is a way. And that is the key reason I am so passionate about the fitness industry and especially about helping you obtain your health goals.

As a personal trainer, I empathize with my clients' turmoil when they talk about the difficulty of trying to make changes in their health. Part of the training I offer is a training of mental attitude. Hearing over and over that there is something wrong with you because your body doesn't match the ideal creates a perception that you are bad in general. I understand how to get through that because I had to do it myself.

Self-destructive behaviors can come from low self-esteem, such

> *You have to embrace yourself before you can change yourself*

as overeating to push down the shame, or avoiding participation in exercise classes because you don't want others to judge you as "too fat" or "too skinny" or even "too awkward."

Low self-esteem and poor body image can even spiral into avoiding relationships or any situation that might mean you have to make yourself vulnerable, even if you know it could eventually create happiness. You essentially block out all of the good things life has to offer because you let the negative image of yourself take over your life. I want to help you delve into your issues, understand them, and move beyond them. You have to embrace yourself before you can change yourself.

Body Image / Self-Image

Body image is defined as the way you view your body as far as attractiveness and overall appearance. Your body image is shaped throughout your life, but especially through your childhood experiences. Comments by your friends and family are often instrumental in having a positive or negative body image.

Self-image is your sense of self, including your body and personality traits such as whether you think you are outgoing, confident, or insecure. It is also defined by how you perceive that others value you.

I am here to affirm that your value as a person is not what the scale says or what the magazines and media tell you that you should be. Both your body image and your self-image need to be realistic and healthy in order for you to be able to make the changes in your lifestyle that will create the fitness and health that you desire.

You need to protect a healthy self-image. If you don't consistently feed your mind positive thoughts about who you are and what you are capable of achieving, you won't be able to get long-lasting fitness results no matter how good the workout and diet programs are. Do you know why? Because if you don't foster a healthy self-image, diet and exercise programs will only be Band-Aids on much deeper and bigger problems.

This wound of a bad self-image and negative body image can be dealt with, though. Start by asking yourself questions that will help you reveal your mental trouble areas. Doing so helps you focus and makes it possible to work on the core problems.

- How do you feel about your body?
- Is the happiness in your day based on what the scale says?
- Are you comfortable discussing some of your insecurities with your close friends or family?
- Do you feel if you are not "perfect" or "better looking" you can't attract a relationship or that you don't deserve one?
- When was the first time you actually felt proud or ashamed of your body?
- Why did you feel that way?
- Are some of your health or nutrition habits designed to punish yourself?

Really dig deep when answering these questions. The more detailed you can be, the greater results you will have.

What you will find by answering these questions are the key motivators—often unconscious—of your behavior and health habits.

When you see yourself being motivated by negative energy, make the effort to change your inner dialogue. For example, if you are thinking "I am so fat" all the time, consciously replace that with "I can make choices that make me healthier every day." Repeat it to yourself often, and over time it becomes your new inner dialogue.

The goal is to be able to be motivated by positive energy so that you can have long-term healthy results.

Society and You

All advertising is designed to hit your insecurities so that you can purchase things to fix yourself. You know, like the picture of the guy with the perfect abs or the girl with the thighs that don't have an ounce of cellulite on them.

But remind yourself that those pictures are airbrushed and digitally enhanced for the specific purpose of attacking your inner core self-value and your self-image in order to take money out of your wallet and put it into the pocket of Company X.

I personally hate this marketing tactic. It certainly gives people the wrong impression about how they should look and feel. I have a friend who works very closely in the "industry of perception," as I like to call it, and he says that everything that they do is to make us believe that we, the general public, are somehow "messed up" and need to be fixed.

I want to challenge you to stop comparing yourself to those photographs in magazines and ad campaigns. It's okay to like how the pictures look and want to strive to achieve similar attributes, but it is not okay to base your self-worth on those pictures.

We are not "messed up" physically but we *are* getting "messed up" mentally by giving up on our own potential when we think we can't measure up to images of body that are illusions.

Instead, the best way to measure your success is to compete against yourself. Know what specific goals you want to achieve. Know why you want to achieve them.

Look at your core issues and face them. Change your inner dialogue. Know that part of the achievement is simply working to better yourself every day. Then focus one hundred percent of your energies on reaching those goals and before you know it you will be there! Healthier in body *and* mind.

How I Can Help You Achieve Your Goals

I'll get you started in chapter one, getting the right structures in place for your new health program and introducing you to the basic concepts we'll be delving into with detail in the following chapters. This will be where we take a baseline of your current fitness level so you know how to move forward.

In the chapter "The Missing Link," I will go over the importance of mental training and how you can use it in your workout regimen to get long-lasting results. I will also go over some exercises that will teach you how to dig into your psyche to get a better understanding of yourself and learn how to change habits that are holding you back from attaining your goals.

In the nutrition chapters I will break down the basics of nutrition so that you can understand what should and shouldn't go into your meals and immediately be able to apply it in your every day life. I will also cover the essential way to put meals together in order to get the results you want.

The chapter on resistance training will cover the basics of repetitions and sets. I'll also go over the most commonly asked questions about resistance training. (Note: whether your goal is to lose weight or increase muscle mass, you *need* to read this chapter.)

The cardio section will cover how long you should do various cardio exercises as well as some of the best ways to get results by using different cardio techniques. I will cover each type of equipment and which ones you should specifically be using to get the results you want.

And finally, in the chapter "Putting It Together," I will discuss how to build your healthy lifestyle by putting all the pieces of the previous chapters together. I not only give you sample workout routines but provide a simple way of building your own workout program. My goal with this chapter is to teach you how to train yourself and how to continue to achieve results.

My big picture goal is to motivate you to make exercising a part of your everyday life. This is why I want to give you a strong foundation in both fitness education—how resistance training, cardio, *and* nutrition work together—*as well as* that added key piece of how to change your mindset to be successful—so that you can live a healthy lifestyle forever.

Whether you are a beginner or a fitness veteran, I wrote this book to help you push to the next level and attain your goals.

As always, be sure that you consult your physician before you start any nutrition and/or exercise program.

Contact Info

www.facebook.com/thefiture

www.twitter.com/thefiture

www.fiture.co

www.youtube.com/gregmarshall17

https://plus.google.com/u/0/116412426702053830049/posts

greg@fiture.co

BODY FIT

CHAPTER ONE

Getting Started

*A journey of a thousand steps
must begin with a single step.*

—Lao Tzu

General Concepts

Nutrition

Nutrition is eating a balanced diet of nutrients to achieve your fitness goals. This is done with a focus on eating the macronutrients—protein, carbohydrates, and fats—while also eating nutrient-dense foods in order to increase energy, maintain a healthy body weight, and live a life full of vitality.

Resistance Training

Resistance training is the use of resistance in the form of body weight, weighted machines, dumbbells, barbells, etc. Resistance training will help increase lean muscle tissue as well as flexibility.

All of the exercises in this text are described in the Exercise Glossary at the back of the book.

Cardiovascular Training

Cardiovascular training, or "cardio," is accomplished by using equipment such as treadmills, stationary bikes, and elliptical machines or by performing body-weight exercises such as swimming, running, and hiking. Cardiovascular training is designed to increase your heart rate. This can provide you with many health benefits such as decreased blood pressure, reduced risk for heart disease, and reduced stress.

Lifestyle

The effects of lifestyle are often overlooked when trying to get fit. There are several factors that play a role in how well your body responds to your workouts. These include sleep, hydration, stress levels, and mental health. Pay close attention to these factors in your life, and work to keep them in an optimal state.

For example, if you are sleep-deprived, your body won't have a chance to recover sufficiently from your workouts. Lack of sleep causes your cortisol levels to increase and puts the body into a catabolic state. Catabolism is a form of destructive metabolism; it inhibits the body from recovery—and inhibits weight loss, if that is your goal.

Time and Intensity

My general rule of thumb is forty minutes of weight training and twenty minutes of cardio.[1] The changes you make in the routine are through varying the exercises and intensity. Increasing intensity—how hard you work your body in a given amount of time—in your workout program is important if you want to see results.

You should not be working out longer than sixty minutes unless you are extremely advanced in your fitness journey, or are competing in certain sports or marathons. If you are going for normal health results, progressively add more work *within* that sixty-minute time frame to get your body to respond. You do this by increasing the intensity of exercises over time: from walking to jogging to running, from a flat surface to a steep incline, and by using resistance training sets like drop sets and super sets that really challenge the muscles. But remember that you should only be increasing your intensity in small increments.

The Dreaded Plateau

Plateaus are something you'll have to contend with from time to time. It occurs when your body no longer responds to the exercises that you are doing. This is one of the main reasons why people don't succeed in their fitness journey. They see the results diminish, so they stop working out. But you can avoid this pitfall by consistently switching up your workout routine.

If we are doing the same exercises day after day and start to see results, the natural inclination is to keep doing the same routine until you get to your goal. The only problem is, the body doesn't work that way. The body adapts to what we give it. Although it seems counterintuitive to change a workout program that is working well for you, this is exactly what will take you to the next level.

How to Avoid Plateaus

I recommend that you don't follow a consistent routine for more than four weeks before making some changes in activity choice and intensity. And certainly, if you are seeing fewer results, that is an indication that it is time to change things up, also.

> *Put 100 percent effort and focus into your program. Constanly challenge yourself.*

The way I explain the plateau to my personal training clients is, I don't train a 180-pound man the same way I train a 130-pound woman, but the *strategy* is the same: switch up your workout program while increasing the intensity. This is true whether you are trying to build muscle mass and get bigger (which is what most men want to do) or build lean muscle tissue and lose body fat (which is what most women want to do).

The best way to get off of a fitness plateau is to completely change your fitness routine and put your body into a "muscle shock" mode. One way to do that is by changing the amount of reps that you do in your workouts. If you usually do sets of 10, switch to doing sets of 15. Or if you usually do two sets of each exercise, increase to three sets. You can also change it up by altering your rest interval. If you usually rest two minutes in between your sets, rest only one minute instead. Put one hundred percent effort and focus into your program. Constantly challenge yourself.

Variety is king, so make sure you don't fall in love with one style of training. Mix it up for the best results. This applies to weight loss just as much as it applies to bodybuilding.

Assess Your Fitness Level

Start by talking to your doctor to make sure that you are able to begin a fitness program. Read this book through and talk to your doctor about how you'd like to incorporate my principles into your life. Continue to check in with your doctor regarding your progress and health during the process.

Assessing your baseline, or starting point, includes measuring body fat, weight, height, body mass index, and your current fitness levels. You will need a body fat tester, a scale, some measuring tape, and a heart rate monitor.

Body Fat

There are a number of highly expensive and scientific means to measuring your body fat level, but the cheapest and easiest ways are to:

- borrow a body fat tester at your local gym or university athletics department,

- purchase a body fat tester online or at a sporting goods store,

- buy a scale that measures body fat,

- pay a personal trainer to do a skin-caliper test, or

- ask a doctor to measure body fat.

Recommended body fat percentages according to the National Academy of Sports Medicine:[2]

Female Fat Percentage

Essential Fat[3]	10—13%	(Percentage of fat required for a woman to maintain her health)
Athletes	14—20%	
Fitness	21—24%	
Acceptable	25—31%	
Obese	32%+	

Male Fat Percentage

Essential Fat[3]	2—5%	(Percentage of fat required for a man to maintain his health)
Athletes	6—13%	
Fitness	14—17%	
Acceptable	18—25%	
Obese	25%+	

Body Mass Index

The body mass index (BMI) is a way to assess your body-fat levels by using your height and weight. It is not the most accurate means of measurement, as it can misinterpret a 200-pound bodybuilder with eight percent body fat as obese, but it helps with an overall understanding of where your body is in accordance with other "average" bodies.

My position on BMI is similar to my beliefs about body weight. I don't want to say that it isn't important, but be sure to look at *all* of your statistics to analyze the success of your program. And remember:

You are assessing how to develop a program *for you*, not anyone else You are assessing a baseline to help you measure your progress, you are *not* assessing your value as a person (more on that later).

BMI = (your weight in pounds x 703) ÷ (your height in inches **x** your height in inches)

For example, if you weigh 120 pounds and are 5 ft. 3 in. (63 in.) tall:

BMI = (120 x 703) ÷ (63 x 63)

which is

84360 ÷ 3969 = 21.3

BMI Statistics[4]

Underweight:	BMI less than 18.5
Normal:	BMI 18.5—24.9
Overweight:	BMI 25—29.9
Obese:	BMI 30 +

Measurements

Some standard measuring points to track your progress are around your:

- Neck
- Upper arm
- Chest
- Hips
- Mid thigh
- Calf

Your measurements will be one of the best gauges of your progress, as body weight can be misleading. You may lose fat and gain muscle and not see a change in the scale, but because muscle is leaner (taking up less volume) than fat, you will see changes in your measurements.

When measuring your body, it is important to have the same person take your measurements every time and/or write down the exact locations where you took your measurements. For example, if you took your measurements for your legs six inches down from your hip, then be sure to mark that down on your progress sheet in order to keep your measuring consistent. A mistake that is made by many trainers and individuals is measuring six inches from the hip one time and then ten inches from the hip another, you may end up with results that aren't relevant to the actual changes in the body shape.

Heart Rate–Baseline Test

The purpose of the heart rate test is to see how well your heart responds to cardiovascular exercise. Before you begin, take your resting pulse.[5] Then, take a ten-minute brisk walk on a treadmill or on a level plane. Afterward, take your pulse again at one-minute intervals for a few minutes (or just until it returns to your resting heart rate). This is your rate (speed) of recovery. The faster your body returns to your resting heart rate, the more conditioned you are.

This will be your baseline and is a great measurement tool. Each day, week, and month you can track your progress. The goal is to have your heart rate recover faster after workouts. That will be the sign that you are getting into better shape.

I'll get into more detail about how to use heart-rate training to tailor your cardio workouts in the cardio chapter.

Workout Attire

What you wear when you work out makes a difference in how well you perform and how motivated you will be. Look at your workout attire as a uniform. If you are going to make a lifestyle change, how you feel is important. You want to make sure that your workout attire is comfortable, helps you perform better, and gets you in the state of mind to push yourself.

Never wear clothes that don't breathe, like jeans, or clothes that aren't appropriate to movement, like dress shirts. Also avoid wearing inappropriate footwear like boots. And leave the jewelry at home, as it may either break off, get dinged, or get lost.

You don't have to spend a lot of money on these items, but I recommend that you don't wear stained, ripped, and worn-out clothing. Feeling good about the way you look when you work out can have just as much of an effect on your productivity as it does in the office. Your workout attire is an investment.

When choosing a workout uniform, be sure to purchase multiple types of clothing and outfits so that they are readily available for you to use each day. You want to minimize the chance of not working out because your uniform is dirty. I would suggest purchasing anywhere from three to six different outfits to match the amount of days that you are going to work out.

The uniform should consist

> *Feeling good about the way you look when you work out can have just as much of an effect on your productivity as it does in the office.*

of comfortably fitting shorts or exercise pants, athletic top, and gym shoes. The shorts or pants should not make you feel self-conscious about your body. Be sure your clothing is neither too baggy nor too tight.

Your workout shoes are the most important things you wear as they will be used on a daily basis. They should fit comfortably and have good soles. Try several different types of gym shoes on to see which ones fit you the best. Do not rely solely on a brand name of shoe. Everyone has differently shaped feet and arches, therefore some shoes will be better for you than others.

Tools for Working Out at Home

It doesn't matter whether you are training at home or at a gym. The only difference between the two is equipment. Weights like dumbbells and high-tech machines are just tools. They are there to help you get results, but they are not the *only* way to get results. So don't mentally limit yourself by thinking that if you don't have these specific tools, it is impossible to get results. On the contrary, you can.

If you are going to work out at home, invest in a jump rope, yoga mat, stopwatch, and resistance bands.

Flooring

Pay attention to the flooring or surface you are on. The reason for this is to avoid putting too much pressure on your joints and tendons. The best flooring to work out on is typically a padded surface or mat because it will absorb more impact than a hard floor such as tile, hard wood, or concrete. Therefore, if you are working out at home and are doing exercises such as squat jumps, invest in a yoga mat or padded mat for the ground or perform them in an area that will be able to absorb impact.

Greg's Tips

- Invest some time reading and re-reading this book as well as finding other educational materials that make understanding the fitness concepts easier and more applicable to your life.

- Understand that this is a lifestyle change and you will not be perfect right away—this is a journey.

- Do not underestimate the small details such as workout attire and carefully tracking where you are now and how you are responding to future workouts as your body becomes more conditioned.

- If you don't get your rest, you don't get results.

- Expect to hit plateaus and have a game plan prepared in advance to motivate yourself through those plateaus.

CHAPTER TWO

The Missing Link: Mental Fitness

Your fitness journey should be every bit spiritual and mental as it is physical.

- G.M.

In this chapter we will talk about what I believe is missing from most workout programs and other fitness advice books: the mental aspect of your fitness goals. Weights, cardio, and nutrition will only get you so far if there are emotions, habits, or feelings holding you back from your true potential.

The tools to reach all of your fitness goals are out there. So why is it that so many people are having a hard time reaching their goals? Let's discover the missing link and a take a leap forward toward changing your life forever.

What Is Mental Training?

Mental training is a core function of success in your fitness journey and in your life. It can be one of the most important tools you have. Mental training requires you to dig deep into yourself to understand why you have certain behaviors. Look at what core emotional issues may be holding you back, focus on improving those mental obstacles, and consciously work to replace negative behaviors with those that help you reach your goals.

If you do the work required—although I know that it can be quite difficult to sift through the basis of negative emotions—you can become not only more fit but see your life change for the better permanently.

Set your mind to support your goals. Change what you tell yourself about behaviors or desires that sabotage your efforts to be healthy. For example, replace the thought of, "I love candy" with "I love feeling healthy and invigorated."

Start to become very conscious of your inner monologue, the way you talk to yourself and the things you say. Find positive mantras that support your goals to replace negative self-talk.

Some of the best athletes, actors, moms and most successful people in the world are successful because they have

> *Strive to bring your best self each and every day. Understand that there will be setbacks, failures, and mental challenges, but you will persevere and come out on top.*

discovered this missing link. They have trained themselves to believe in their goals and to work as hard as they can and dedicate their life to being the best at what they do.

Like these people, strive to bring your best self each and every day. Understand that there will be setbacks, failures, and mental challenges, but you will persevere and come out on top.

It could be, though, that you have some serious issues to grapple with or that you are in such a mental rut with negativity that you need to seek out a counselor, psychologist, or psychiatrist to help you work through the process. Don't be afraid to do so. If you really want to become healthy, the mental aspect is crucial.

Discovering Your "Why"

In order to truly reach your potential and stay motivated for a sustainable amount of time, you must understand your "Why." Why do you want to better yourself? What motivates you? It's hard to stay motivated just by *telling yourself that you should* do better or be better—sometimes that can even be harmful. Instead, strike to your core and *feel* the reasons *why* you are doing what you are doing. And then take the time to figure out your "Why": why you want to better yourself.

It can be hard, but allow your emotions to get involved in this process to get the maximum results. We are driven to do things by emotion. First, understand the emotion that has kept you from attaining your goals or the emotions that support negative behaviors. Then you need to give yourself a strong emotional connection as to why you want to change your behaviors.

Ask Yourself:

- Who was your role model growing up? And why?
- Who is your role model currently? And why?
- What makes you feel the most positive about yourself?
- What makes you feel negative and unmotivated?
- What kind of legacy do you want to leave?
- With what kind of people do you associate yourself?
- With whom do you *want* to associate yourself?
- Why are you going to make a permanent change in your life?

Stories of "Why"

As a personal trainer, I've heard a lot of people's reasons why they want to get in better physical shape. Often, coming to terms with making their bodies physically healthy is also a process of working through emotional issues so that they are mentally healthy, too.

I've had several clients like Jim,[1] who said he was made fun of in school as "the fat kid." That experience created insecurities that he noticed had transferred into other aspects of his life as he grew into adulthood. Jim felt like he was coming up short in life. He noticed his eating habits and life habits were a form of self-punishment for not living up to what others—and he—thought he should be. He wanted to make a change in his life and that is "why" Jim asked for help.

Karrie grew up in an extended family of which many members

were obese. Heart disease, diabetes, and joint pain were common ailments in her family. Karrie was moved to action by watching her family members deal with poor self-esteem due to their poor physical health. She recognized how obesity

You deserve to take care of yourself. You deserve time that you spend on your health. And I believe in your ability to achieve your goals. You can better your health and your life. Let's work together as a team.

negatively affected every aspect of her family members' lives. She decided that she wanted to stop the trend by watching her own health carefully. She wanted to be a good role model to her children, as well as to her family members who were struggling with their health. This was Karrie's "Why."

When Jennifer came in for her first appointment with me it was clear she had lost hope in her life and herself. Her husband had filed for a divorce, she had a teenage daughter, and she was more than 100 pounds overweight. She said that she felt helpless and came to me because she needed help and wanted to get control of her life again.

Jennifer said she wanted to train with me, but in the middle of the meeting, she suddenly told me she couldn't afford a personal trainer and walked away. I felt really badly because I could see the pain in Jennifer's face and I desperately wanted to help her achieve her goals. I wanted to help her get her life back.

The next day Jennifer came back into the gym. With tears in

her eyes, she said that she could afford to work with me but that she was scared to commit because she was afraid to fail. What an emotional moment it was for both of us as she let out so much of the sorrow and frustration that she had kept bottled inside. "I need to start training with you, though, because I don't know what else to do," she said.

What I told her, I tell you: You deserve to take care of yourself. You deserve the time that you will spend on your health. And I believe in your ability to achieve your goals. You can better your health and your life. Let's work together as a team.

Jennifer and I took some time to discover her "Why." She wanted to prove to herself that she could accomplish this goal of getting back into shape and rediscovering herself. She not only wanted it for herself but for her daughter. She wanted to be a good role model and be sure that her daughter had healthy footsteps in which to follow.

> *I want to be here to tell you every day that you deserve to be happy and can achieve your goals.*

As Jennifer and I worked out together, I listened as she talked out some of her issues and began the process of healing. I gave her encouragement every day to believe in herself. She got back into hobbies that she had once loved, and over time, Jennifer reached her goals.

Jim, Karrie, and Jennifer are parts of *my* "Why": why I love this job. To see people make changes that increase the vitality, health, quality, and, probably, length of their lives is why I work as a personal trainer. It is also why I wanted to write this book.

I want to be here to tell *you* every day that you deserve to be happy and you can achieve your goals. And I want to break down the process so that I can help you figure out how to do it.

Your Fitness Journal

You can't improve what you don't consciously and consistently measure and analyze. To improve yourself, you must know your self at your core. You must understand what drives you to feel happy, sad, angry, or fulfilled. This will require some serious self-reflection on your part.

A daily fitness journal can help you discover trends in your behavior so that you can make changes and eliminate self-sabotage. This fitness journal will include three sections: a food journal (more on that in the nutrition chapter), a workout journal (tracking both your activities and your weight/measurements), and a personal journal. In the personal journal section I want you to look back into your childhood and write about the events that have helped shape who you are today.

Think about and write down the events that made you happy and loved and cared for. Also write down the events that have caused you to feel sad or insecure. I want you to write these events down in as much detail as possible including who was there, why you felt the way you did, what you liked or disliked about the event, and what environment you were in.

Consistently write through these events all the way up to your life today. Put some serious thought and effort into understanding how these various events have shaped your personal daily habits in life: exercise, parenting, work habits, and relationships. You may be surprised what you learn about yourself.

Being conscious of your activities and what motivates you to make your choices will keep you away from autopilot living. That's when you can start to make the necessary adjustments to create the exact environment you need to succeed.

Sara's Story

One of my clients, Sara, said that every time she accomplished something important, her family would go out to eat to celebrate. This made her feel really happy and connected with her family. It made her feel loved.

Celebrating with food is a common experience and hits upon a core emotion that we humans have, which is to feel love from people that we care about immensely.

Those were the times that Sara valued and cherished the most, to feel the endorphin rush of accomplishing a goal as well as the acceptance of her family. These good feelings were connected to food for her.

Sara grew older and started a family. She became extremely busy with her kids and household. She was a very loving and caring mom but always put the family and everyone else's needs first. In doing so, she forgot to take care of herself.

While she got great fulfillment from being a mother, she would get tired and worn out. So when the kids were asleep and her husband was at work, she would turn to food—the thing that she associated with love and positive emotions—to make her feel better.

The food comforted her, but she started to gain weight. So she decided that she wanted to do something for herself. Sara purchased a gym membership and worked with a personal trainer. She went faithfully, but she noticed that for some reason she was just not getting the results that she wanted.

We analyzed her workouts and she was training the right way. We analyzed her cardio workouts and she was performing those correctly as well. She seemed to be doing everything right.

But when we analyzed Sara's nutrition, she was struggling to eat healthfully each day and stick to a nutrition plan. She could not figure out why she could be so disciplined with her workouts but seemed to lack the will power to control her eating habits. This started to affect Sara's self-esteem and self-worth. She was extremely frustrated.

Using the fitness journal to record the emotions behind her eating gave us insight into what was going wrong. Sara's problem wasn't will power, but habit and association. When she felt lonely, she would use food to bring her a sense of satisfaction and the feeling of love she mentally connected with food.

I knew that if we could satisfy that need for human support and interaction that Sara craved, she would be able to successfully create and stick to our nutrition plan. So instead of making her diet more strict, we came up with some different solutions. Sara and I set up a goal to enrich her emotional relationship with her husband. She needed to let him know that he was not failing as a husband, but that she had specific needs that he was capable of meeting that would help her improve her life. Also, Sara had to schedule time out of the week for herself. She started taking a girl's night out, to develop deeper and more meaningful relationships with her friends. This gave her a special time and place to recharge that she could look forward to.

After making some of these changes, Sara was not only better able to meet her nutritional goals, but her life became more fulfilled and balanced. And from this, she was able to break through her fitness plateau.

The purpose of sharing this story with you is to challenge you to think outside of the box. It may not be a lack of will power keeping you from reaching your goals, but deeper emotional issues that need to be addressed.

What Do You Want From Life?

Defining what you want from life is extremely important in the goal-setting process. Not knowing where you are going is the beginning of a frustrating journey. By clearly identifying what you want to accomplish, you can not only put together a game plan, but you can also begin to get yourself excited about your destination. Excitement and motivation come from believing you have a brighter future ahead of you. You have to believe.

This is the beginning of a life-changing process—making the decision to better yourself—and most people get excited about the opportunities that lay ahead. The thoughts of being a healthier you should give you the initial motivation that you will need.

If, however, you are holding back due to fear of not reaching your goals, you can get excited by asking yourself:

- How will I feel about myself when I reach a goal that I set out to achieve?

- How much more confident will I feel when I want to go swimming or go to the beach?
- How great will it feel to shop for the clothes that I want instead of settling for clothes that I fit into?
- What exact date do I want to weigh my goal weight?
- What benchmarks can I celebrate along my way to reaching my big-picture goal?

Creating Your Action Plan

Once you discover your "Why," your job is to list your fitness goals and tie them to your "Why."

By keeping this line of thinking in mind as you do your training activities, you will see a significant difference in your motivation and success. Your actions will have meaning. It will become more than just going through the motions of a workout program and you will be able to stick to your program more than you ever have in the past.

You *will* go through the ups and downs of hitting plateaus and setbacks. If you know your "Why," you will have the reason to keep going and push through to the other side.

First, start the fitness journal I described earlier in the chapter. In the front of the book, or on a bookmark, write *MY "WHY"* and list three to five main motivating factors that drive you to succeed. Before you write in your journal each day I want you to review your "Why."

Second, add photos that symbolize your "Why." Choose the pictures wisely. Make sure they emotionally resonate for you. The pictures should visually depict the feelings that are most important to you and serve as a constant reminder about why you are changing your lifestyle. You can put these in the front of your journal, or create a vision board—a place your "Why" pictures are posted that you can see every day.

> *Change is hard, but your "Why" will pull you through.*

Third, I want you to find a partner or a support group to whom you are accountable. This partner should remind you of your goals and, most importantly, "Why" they are important to you. The partner you choose must be someone who is supportive and compassionate, but not afraid to tell you the truth and speak candidly. Choose this person carefully as his or her support and ability to make you accountable for your actions can be key to taking your fitness to the next level.

Fourth, set up a reward system that will motivate you and provide the positive reinforcement that you need. This is an often-overlooked part of a fitness program and it is easy to get caught in the trap of setting "moving targets" as goals. For example, if you promise to buy a new pair of shoes after you reach ten pounds, and the first ten pounds comes off easily, don't wait until you lose fifteen pounds to buy the shoes. Reward yourself and set a new goal. The reward—especially if it is a tangible item or an experience—will be another visual reminder of your accomplishment and the need to keep going.

Change is hard, but your "Why" will pull you through.

Goal Setting: The SMART Principle[2]

I've adapted Paul J. Meyer's SMART goal characteristics to relate to body health changes. Use this as a general guideline for reaching your fitness goals.

Specific:

Be specific about what you want to achieve. Have short-term and long-term goals. For example, a short-term goal would be to lose ten pounds, a long-term goal to lose thirty.

Measurable:

Document your progress in the workout section of your journal so you can measure your success. For example, weigh yourself every two weeks.

Actionable:

Have a specific plan in place as to what your workout will consist of each day and what you will eat each day. Make sure you prepare everything in advance so that there are no excuses to back out.

Realistic:

Keep your goals in line with what is both possible and healthy. Generally speaking, two pounds a week is a healthy weight-loss goal. Depending on how much you have to lose, the first couple of weeks you may see more weight loss. On the other hand, as muscle is built, you may even see weight gains the first couple of weeks. Stick with it, and the loss should start to regulate.

Time-bound:

Give yourself a deadline to meet your short-term and long-term goals. Nothing motivates like a deadline.

Fitness Setbacks

Oftentimes we are afraid to set goals using the SMART principle because we are inherently afraid to fail. There is a subconscious thought that holds us back: *If I hold myself accountable to a goal, what happens if I don't reach it?*

When setting goals, you have to understand that there *will* be setbacks and failures. You must be realistic. No one who has achieved worthwhile goals gets there easily. The road to success isn't straight and smooth. How you handle the bumps on the road to your goal will become the measure of how successful you will be in seeing it through to the end.

Think of setbacks as a test of how badly you want it.

It is easy and normal to feel frustrated when your progress slows. Some people give themselves the excuse that something is wrong with them genetically. But it is just the science of how you are going to break out of the plateau that matters. Becoming educated so that you know how to adjust your actions, and knowing that you must have patience during plateaus as you adjust, will help you get through.

How To Handle Fitness Setbacks

Before you get too worked up about a plateau, make sure you are doing the correct exercises and that you are doing them correctly. Then look at your training regimen and the data you've kept on your activities to see if you are changing your workouts enough. See if your intensity is lagging; consider whether you are giving your best effort in your workouts. Be brutally honest with yourself and use the reality principle. You may have a fear looming in your head that prevents you from giving it your full effort.

In the personal part of your fitness journal, create a list of some of the setbacks that you are experiencing. When you write down the setbacks and problems, you will be controlling the setback instead of letting the setback control you. Isolate each setback and come up with at least five different solutions to the problem. By having more than one solution you can try several strategies to see which one works the best for you.

Create a plan for how you will overcome various setbacks, then consider asking a fitness professional for his or her opinion. Also, find someone who works out regularly in a gym and ask them their opinion about your plan. Go online to a communication platform such as fitocracy.com or join the fitness communities

The road to success isn't straight and smooth. How you handle the bumps on the road to your goal will become the measure of how successful you will be in seeing it through to the end.

on tumblr.com and ask the audience what their opinions are. Write down the feedback you get.

Look over all of the responses you received to see where there are similarities. That is where you should start. Formulate a plan based on that.

Mental Exercises for Dealing with Setbacks

Remember to give yourself some credit for the effort you are putting in. The effort is the success. If you put too much pressure on yourself to hit your goals you will probably end up unhappy. Always maintain the attitude that you can laugh at any situation and don't take yourself too seriously. Be patient.

Another way to deal with a setback is to give yourself a mental break and focus more on other aspects of your life for a short period of time. This does not mean to quit your workout program, but rather keep exercising and tweaking your workouts while simultaneously focusing more of your mental energy on your work or relationships.

Have multiple life goals outside of your fitness goals. This allows you to continue getting positive reinforcement from another area of your life when your fitness is hitting a plateau.

Focus on the positives of what you are doing and the results that you have already achieved. In our quest to be successful it is easy to forget the success already obtained along the journey. Don't discount it. It matters. Nothing is too small of a victory. Celebrate the fact that you are even striving toward a fitness goal. Celebrate that you are exercising regularly. Be proud when you eat one healthy meal in a day. These are different ways to keep a positive outlook on your journey and feel like you are progressing.

In our quest to be successful it is easy to forget the success already obtained along the journey. Don't discount it. It matters.

Read a book on having a positive attitude. These books can serve a great purpose and give you motivation when you are feeling down. A book is also a way to slow down a racing mind and to focus your energies on something other than your obstacles. Listen to motivational speeches in your car or on your mp3 player. Sometimes hearing positive reinforcement come from someone else—anyone else—can make a real difference.

Find a friend who will listen to your struggle. Sometimes all you need to do is express that bottled up disappointment in order to start fresh again. This is a great way to also bond with a friend or a loved one who can support you on your journey. They may become the one to give you that push you need when you feel like giving up. And instead of going out for ice cream to talk about it, talk it over during a brisk walk. You'll feel twice as good at the end.

Greg's Tips

- Discover and define your "Why."

- Study positive attitude and thinking every day.

- Keep a detailed fitness journal to log your workouts, nutrition, and feelings.

- Define what makes you happy and what makes you unhappy.

- Write a detailed page on what you want your life to be.

- Have fun with your journey and keep things light.

- When you feel like you can't do it, just remember your "Why." This is more than just fitness, this is your life.

CHAPTER THREE

Nutrition: Part I

"Let food be thy medicine and medicine be thy food."

—Hippocrates

Nutrition is the fundamental key to losing weight and having more energy. I cannot stress enough that if you are looking to make a real, sustainable lifestyle change, one of the most important things you can do for yourself is to educate yourself about what proteins, carbohydrates, and fats are, and how they work in the body. This will be the best investment of your time if you want to reach and maintain fitness targets.

The Basics of Nutrition

To better understand nutrition, it's essential to understand what makes up the food you eat. The basic building blocks of nutrition are proteins, carbohydrates, fats, and water. You want to combine protein, carbs, and fat in every meal. For vitamins and minerals you need fruits and vegetables. This combination provides more sustainable energy and helps keep your body in a fat-burning zone for longer durations of time.

Water

Water is an essential and often overlooked nutrient in our body. Almost two-thirds of our bodies are water. While much of nutrition discussions these days are focused on low-carb plans or protein intake and vitamins, we forget that the most important nutrient of all is water. Just increasing your water intake will allow your body to utilize your food and supplements more efficiently.

A lot of times when people think they are feeling hungry, what the body is really craving is water. Try drinking a glass or two of water next time you think you are hungry and wait fifteen to twenty minutes to see whether you feel satiated or not.

Most people don't drink enough—and watch out, because sodas don't count, they actually cause dehydration. When you do drink enough water you will notice an increase in energy and focus.

Water is especially important when you are increasing energy output. In my experience, if you are even the slightest bit dehydrated during and after your workout, you will not recover as quickly.

Water helps to stimulate your metabolism and aids in the removal of toxins in the body. You can absolutely trust your instincts as to how thirsty you are—don't drink so much you feel sick. But the following guidelines are a great reference point and helpful if you are a beginner.

A full glass of water is eight ounces. Each day you should drink eight to twelve glasses (eight-ounce sized) of water— depending on your build, workouts, and environment (such as heat, humidity, and/or altitude). As part of this daily total, I recommend:

- Drink two or three full glasses of water (total = sixteen to twenty-four ounces) two to three hours before your exercise.

- Drink a half to a full glass of water (four to eight ounces) every fifteen to twenty minutes during your workout to stay properly hydrated. You may need more or less based on how warm the weather is and how much you weigh. But generally speaking, during a one-hour workout you should drink one-and-a-half to four glasses of water (twelve to thirty-two ounces).

- Drink enough water after your workout that you feel satiated.

If, in spite of this, you are still feeling dehydrated, weigh yourself before and after you workout, and drink one-half to two-thirds of a glass (four to six ounces) of water following your workout per pound that you lost.

Water is the best way to get your body hydrated but if you end up losing a lot of salt during your workouts (and you can tell by an intensely salty taste of your sweat or salt stains on your clothes) then you may need to drink a sports drink that has electrolytes. But be careful, sports drinks have a lot of sugar, so stick to just one sports drink per day—especially if you are a beginner or trying to lose weight. Sip it during your work out and finish it immediately after you exercise.

Protein

Protein is found in foods such as chicken, fish, lean beef, and egg whites. Each gram of protein equals four calories. For example, if you have twenty grams of protein you would consume eighty calories.

Protein is a useful source of energy. You should eat eight-tenths to one gram of protein per pound of body weight per day. For example, if you weigh 120 pounds you would eat between 96 and 120 grams of protein total per day. This food staple has multiple functions in the body that make it a necessity for healthy living.

If you are specifically looking to bulk up, or increase muscle mass, I would increase that amount. One to one and a half grams of protein per pound of body weight per day is ideal.

If you are specifically looking to tone up, try to get one gram of protein per pound of body weight each day and make sure it is lean protein (best: chicken, fish, turkey; avoid: red meat and pork).

Protein:

- helps to build and repair muscles in your body. (When you exercise you cause minute tears in your muscles. Protein helps repair those tears. This is what makes you stronger.)

- stimulates your metabolism.
- repairs, builds, and maintains the body's cells—including regenerating healthy hair, skin, bones, and fingernails.
- supports main organ function, such as regulating the digestive process.
- creates antibodies that help fight infections.

Complete Proteins:

Proteins that provide the essential amino acids to help repair and build muscle fiber. Complete proteins are found in animal meat such as chicken, fish, and beef.

Incomplete Proteins:

Proteins from plants and legumes such as beans, rice, tofu, and certain vegetables. These provide lower amounts of protein per gram and should be combined together in order to provide a meal higher in protein, such as rice and beans. Incomplete proteins are also higher in carbohydrate content than complete proteins. Vegetarian and vegan diets typically consist of these proteins.

Vegetarian/Vegan Options

Vegetarians and vegans can have a more difficult time obtaining the protein that they need because of the incomplete proteins that make up most of their diet. Drinking vegan-based protein shakes, increasing the number of meals per day, and combining a wider array of incomplete proteins in each meal can help.

Too Much of a Good Thing

Too much protein can cause extra stress on the kidneys and liver, which are the body's main filtering systems. The last thing you want to do is put too much stress on organs that get rid of the body's toxins.

Some excess protein in our diets can be converted and stored as fat. Since many animal proteins are high in saturated fats, use them in moderation to prevent high blood pressure and heart disease.

Protein-Rich Foods

In order to make the healthiest protein choices, look for the leanest cuts of meat. Red meats tend to be higher in saturated fat than white meats like fish and chicken. Fish is also higher in healthy fats, which we will discuss later.

Servings and Protein Content[1]

Animal:

- Chicken/turkey breast, 3.5 ounce serving = 30 grams
- Chicken Thigh = 10 grams
- Beef (most cuts) = 7 grams per ounce
- Hamburger patty, 4 ounces = 28 grams
- Egg = 6 grams
- Fish fillets (most) = 6 grams per ounce
- Tuna fish, 7 grams per ounce

Dairy:

- Low-fat cheese stick = 6 grams per ounce
- Cottage cheese, ½ cup = 15 grams
- Milk (get lowest fat content you can handle), 1 cup = 8 grams
- Soy Milk, 1 cup = 6—10 grams
- Yogurt (reduced sugar), 1 cup = 8—12 grams

Vegetable:

- Beans, cooked (black, pinto, lentils, etc.) = 7—10 g per half cup

Nuts and Seeds:

- Peanut butter, 2 tablespoons = 8 grams
- Almonds, ¼ cup = 8 grams
- Peanuts, ¼ cup = 9 grams
- Cashews, ¼ cup = 5 grams
- Pecans, ¼ cup = 2.5 grams
- Sunflower seeds, ¼ cup = 6 grams
- Pumpkin seeds, ¼ cup = 8 grams
- Flax seeds, ¼ cup = 8 grams

Supplements:

- Whey Protein Powder, 1 scoop = 20—30 grams
- Soy Protein Powder, 1 scoop = 20—30 grams

Protein Supplements

Protein supplements are usually found in powders and shakes. Check first with your doctor, but protein supplements can be used if you need help getting your daily requirement of protein. As we said earlier, getting enough protein is necessary for building muscle, and muscle speeds metabolism. (This is how protein shakes can indirectly help you lose weight.)

If you struggle with cooking and have difficulty preparing meals in advance, it is better to have a protein shake than eat fast food or end up not eating at all. But it must be said, while protein shakes are great for supplementing the diet, there is nothing better for your body than natural whole foods. The body can utilize real food much better than a supplement. If you have an option, eat the real thing.

Two of the most commonly used protein shakes are whey protein and casein protein. The differences of the two are how fast the body utilizes them and what they offer specifically towards your goals.

Whey Protein:

Protein full of amino acids, which are important for building muscle and speeding recovery. It is absorbed quickly, which helps the body synthesize the protein well. Whey protein may also help boost the immune system in the body.

The best times to take whey protein shakes is about an hour before and immediately after your workout.

Casein Protein:

A slower digesting protein. It keeps the body from going into a catabolic (muscle-wasting) state that otherwise occurs when you don't eat for a sustained period of time, such as during sleeping. Thus, this is good to ingest in the evening.

Casein protein also provides some amino acids and is a great source of dairy calcium. The best way to use casein protein is to combine it with your meals—especially with whole food proteins—and at dinner.

Note that whey and casein protein are both derived from milk. (In fact, 80 percent of the protein found in milk is casein protein and the remaining 20 percent is whey.) So if you are lactose intolerant, like I am, these probably aren't good choices for you.

You can use soy protein or rice protein instead. That is what I like to use for my protein shakes. Another consideration is a beef protein powder that has recently come to the market. While these don't work exactly as whey and casein do respectively, they are options for getting that protein boost.

Your local health food store will usually carry many different types of protein powders based on your needs. Ask for help if you have digestive problems with certain types of protein shakes. And talk to your doctor about using them.

The key factor in using such shakes is maintaining a regular workout program and a healthy diet.

Carbohydrates

Carbohydrates are sugars. They are your body's main source of energy. Each gram of carbohydrate equals four calories. Carbohydrates come from breads, pastas, oats, grains, fruits, and vegetables.

Not all carbs are created equal. The carbs that you will want to base most of your diet on will be quality carbs such as whole grains—like wheat and oats—and, of course, fruits and vegetables. Generally speaking, fruits are higher in carbohydrates than vegetables, as the fructose in them that makes them sweet is a sugar. Potatoes and corn, though, are very high in sugar.

Eat a steady flow of carbohydrates throughout the day, but frontload the larger portions of carbohydrates in the early part of the day so that your body can utilize them instead of storing them. This is why it is good to eat fruit in the morning and vegetables in the evening.

Do *not* be afraid to eat carbohydrates! But you should track and measure the amount of carbs that your body needs based on how energetic you feel. Pay attention to how sustained your energy levels are throughout the day. Do you feel like you can focus all day and that you have the energy to accomplish your necessary daily tasks? If not, look at how you are putting your meals together and make sure they are balanced. (More on this in Nutrition: Part II.)

People who are looking to lose weight and tone up should choose complex carbohydrates and decrease their intake by about half. If you normally eat a cup of rice at a meal, replace it with a half-cup. If you need to make up calories, do so using protein and/or non-starchy (low-carb) vegetables.

Simple vs. Complex Carbohydrates

Simple Carbohydrates:

Carbohydrates that are burned quickly and spike your insulin and blood sugar levels, while complex carbohydrates burn more slowly, giving you lasting energy.

Simple carbohydrates are found in foods mostly made up of sugar. An example would be fruit juices (natural sugars) and soft drinks (refined sugars). Simple carbohydrates can have their place in the diet, but they can increase body fat, decrease long-term energy, and cause mood swings. Excess simple carbohydrates in the diet are linked with diabetes, high blood pressure, heart disease, and obesity.

There are optimal times to consume simple sugars. Combined with a protein and eaten after your workout, a simple sugar can kick start your body's recovery process. But overall, I would suggest you eat whole fruit after your workout or the healthiest option of carbohydrates you can find.

In fact, simple sugars in your diet should be replaced as often as possible by whole fruits (not juices), whole (brown) grains, oats, vegetables, or water.

Simple Sugars:

- Cakes/pastries
- Candy
- Cookies
- Doughnuts

- Soda

- Syrups

- White rice, white pasta

Refined sugars do not contain any nutrients or vitamins. They are empty calories.

Complex carbohydrates:

Carbohydrates that should be the majority of your carbohydrate intake. They are a source of long-lasting energy and keep your blood sugar stable. Complex carbohydrates come from whole grains, and the pastas, rice, and breads that are made from them. Simply put, complex carbs tend to be brown foods while refined sugars tend to be white foods. Choose brown.

Complex Carbohydrates[2]:

(One carbohydrate serving = 15 grams)

One serving of bread, rice, or cereal:

- 1/2 cup cooked oatmeal
- 1 slice of bread
- 1/2 small bagel
- 1/3 cup cooked pasta or rice
- 3 cups popped popcorn
- 3/4 cup unsweetened cereal
- 6 Saltine crackers

One serving of fruit:

- 15 small grapes
- 1 small (four-inch) banana
- 2 tablespoons raisins
- 3/4 cup berries
- 1 cup cantaloupe or other melon
- 1/2 cup fruit juice (fresh squeezed or store bought)
- 1 small apple

One serving of milk:

- 1 cup milk, nonfat or low-fat
- 1 cup plain yogurt, nonfat or low-fat

Note: Cheese, including cottage cheese, is counted as a protein serving, not a carbohydrate; whereas milk is a complex carbohydrate that also provides a good source of protein.

One serving of dessert or sweets:

- 1/3 of a slice of apple pie (1 slice=1/6 of 8-inch pie)
- 1/2 cup ice cream
- 3 ounces soda pop (1/3 of small can)
- 5 vanilla wafers
- 1 tablespoon honey or sugar

One serving of starchy vegetables:

- 1/2 cup or 1 small ear of corn
- 1/2 cup cooked lentils or dried beans

- 1/2 cup green peas
- 3-inch potato

Fats[3]

Fats are calorie dense and give you a sense of fullness or satiety. Fats are important for regulating the body's natural hormone system. If your diet is too low in fat, you will not be able to utilize its benefit in changing your body's composition. Like carbohydrates, fats have a bad reputation. It seems logical that if you eat fat you will get fat, but it's not necessarily true. It depends *how much* and *what kinds* of fats you are eating.

There are differences in the fat from avocados, which is a healthy fat (monounsaturated), and the fats that come from a doughnut (saturated and trans fats). The fats that come from the two sources do two separate things. Monounsaturated fat adds *value* to your diet and actually helps with nutrition and loss of body fat. There are also good fats like polyunsaturated fats. On the other hand, saturated fat and trans fat *add more body fat* while clogging your arteries.

Total fat:[4]

Limit total fat intake to 20 to 35 percent of your daily calories. Based on a diet of 2,000 calories per day, this amounts to about 44 to 78 grams of fat per day. But your caloric needs may differ.

Healthy Fats[5]

Monounsaturated and polyunsaturated fats play a key role in absorbing vitamins such as A, D, E, and K. Those specific vitamins are considered fat soluble, which means the body cannot utilize them without dietary fat. While these fats are higher in calories per gram than other kinds of foods, they should be in your diet—but stay within your total fat allowance.

Monounsaturated fats

decrease the risk for heart disease and improve levels of cholesterol. These types of fats are also good at stabilizing blood sugar levels when they are ingested with carbohydrates and protein. This can be beneficial for diabetics or people who are trying to lose body fat.

Some foods high in monounsaturated fats are: peanut butter, olives, olive oil, avocados, poultry, and nuts.

Polyunsaturated fats

can help lower your risk for Type 2 Diabetes and heart disease by helping to improve blood cholesterol levels.

Polyunsaturated fats are found in foods such as vegetable oils (flaxseed, safflower, corn, soy, cottonseed, and sunflower), peanut oil, poultry fish, flaxseed oil, seeds, and nuts—especially walnuts.

Omega-3 Fatty Acids:

These acids are found in fatty, cold-water fish (such as salmon, mackerel and herring), ground flaxseed, flax oil, and walnuts. Omega-3 fat is one of the polyunsaturated fats that seem to help reduce the chances of developing coronary artery disease.

No specific amount of omega-3 fats is recommended, but it goes without saying that you should try to get more of your total fat intake from healthy fats than from unhealthy fats.

Unhealthy Fats

Saturated Fat:

Fats that clog up the arteries and can cause health problems such as cardiovascular disease and high blood pressure. Whole milk, red meat, french fries, cookies, fast food, and desserts are all high in saturated fats—as are cheese, pizza, and animal products, such as fried chicken dishes, sausage, hot dogs, bacon, and ribs. Other sources: lard, butter, and tropical oils like coconut and palm.

Limit saturated fat intake to no more than 10 percent of your total calories (about 22 grams, based on a 2,000-calorie-per-day diet), or, to reduce risk of heart disease, try to limit it to 7 percent (about 15 grams, based on a 2,000-calorie-per-day diet).[6] Your intake should be lower if you are trying to tone up and/or lose weight or have a lower calorie diet.

Trans Fat:

Trans fats are, in my opinion, the least healthy of all because it hardens arteries, which impedes circulation. Most trans fats come from processed foods or any food that is mass-produced. Trans fat is popular in restaurants and processed food companies because it helps keep the food from spoiling. It is found in margarines, snack foods, and prepared desserts.

It's difficult to eliminate all trans fats because there are some that are naturally occurring in meat and dairy foods. Obviously, trans fat in a glass of whole milk is a better choice than getting it from processed food, but either way the American Heart Association recommends limiting trans fat to no more than 1 percent of your total daily calories.[7] For most people, this is less than two grams a day.

Cholesterol:

Your cholesterol intake should be less than 300 milligrams a day—less than 200 milligrams a day if you're at high risk of cardiovascular disease. Cholesterol is found in eggs and egg dishes, chicken dishes, beef dishes, and hamburgers. Other sources: seafood, dairy products, lard, and butter.

Fruits and Vegetables

Fruits and vegetables are a vital part to overall fitness because they are not only a healthy energy source, but also provide critical antioxidants, which are important for helping the body regenerate. An easy way to increase antioxidants in your diet is to choose a variety of colors of fruits and vegetables. The more variety, the more vitamins and minerals your body has to feed your cells and keep you feeling healthy. Choose a fruit or vegetable to complement each meal. They will also help with digestion.

A Word about Sauces and Dressings

When eating salads and making sandwiches, keep the sauces and dressings to a minimum. Use sauces to add flavor, but stay disciplined by using 2 tablespoons maximum. Sauces are like silent calories—they add up quickly. Here are some ideas for healthier sauce and dressing options:

- Garlic powder
- Hot sauce (watch for sodium content)
- Ketchup, organic (watch sugar content; avoid those with corn syrup)
- Low-fat ranch dressing
- Mustard, regular or spicy (watch for sodium content)
- Olive oil
- Olive oil cooking spray
- Olive oil and vinegar
- Oregano
- Raspberry vinaigrette

- Red pepper flakes

- Reduced-fat mayo with olive oil

- Salsa (watch for sodium content)

- Vinegar

Snacks

Eating often is crucial in any weight-control diet and fitness regimen. Frequent but controlled meals keep your metabolism running at its peak efficiency. Snacks should be fun and offer variety.

Keep portions small. To keep it simple, I advise my clients to keep solid food snacks to about the size of their closed fist. Liquid snacks should be eight to 12 ounces.

I recommend two or three snacks per day in addition to three meals.

Change up your snacks so you can get a variety of flavors and nutrients while simultaneously being able to develop good lifestyle habits.

This list is just an example of some great options. Get creative!

- Almonds or nuts

- Apples with peanut butter

- Beef jerky, low sodium

- Bran (or high-fiber) cereal, handful, dry

- Celery sticks with peanut butter

- Cheese stick, low-fat

- Chocolate milk

- Fiber bar

- Frozen fruit

- Fruit smoothie with protein powder

- Fruit, one bowl

- Fruit juice (although eating the actual fruit is better; try for organic, and also look for juice with added protein)

- Meal-replacement shake

- Oat cereal, handful, dry

- Oatmeal mixed with frozen fruit

- Protein shake, smoothie, or bar

- Salad: romaine lettuce or spinach with low-calorie, low-sodium dressing of 2 tablespoons or less

- Trail mix (keep it to a smaller bag so sugar content is not too high)

- Turkey or tuna fish sandwich on whole wheat bread, HALF

- Turkey and cheese wrap with whole-wheat tortilla

- Vegetables, one bowl

- Yogurt (low sugar) cup with granola

Supplements

Supplements can be added to your nutrition program but they are just that: *supplementary* to a good died. Don't rely on them too much. Get your nutrition from whole foods first, supplements second. Supplements can help you reach your goals but stick with the ones that have been highly researched and have some data backing them up.

There are pros and cons to using supplements, and most are not regulated by the Food and Drug Administration, so choose wisely before purchasing them.

In addition to the protein supplements that I recommended earlier in this chapter, I have used each one of the following supplements personally as well as suggested many of these to clients.

Research the brands and check with your doctor about both the supplement itself and how much you are interested in taking.

- BCAA supplements—used for recovery and keeping the body in an anabolic state
- Casein protein—protein shake derived from milk; great for preventing a catabolic state (muscle wasting)
- Creatine—used for ATP production (energy); it helps to replace the energy that is used when you weight lift or do sprinting activities, so you can train at higher intensities
- Egg protein—eggs are considered one of the most efficiently absorbed proteins available
- Essential fatty acids—multiple sources of fats that help regulate hormones and increase fat burn

- Flaxseed oil—source of healthy fat that can help to regulate hormones and increase fat burn
- Glucosamine and chondroitin—help with lubricating joints and are helpful for people who suffer from stiffness
- Glutamine—amino acid used specifically to help with muscle recovery; a natural precursor to human growth hormone
- Green tea—great for fat loss and adding antioxidants into your diet; can aid recovery after a workout
- Multivitamin—helps to balance out nutritional deficiencies
- Omega 3-6-9 oil—fish oils that help the body burn fat, regulate hormones, and may aid cognitive function
- Plant protein—protein shake for vegans and vegetarians
- Protein bars—quick snack used to replace granola bars with higher protein content
- Rice protein—protein shake that is good for lactose-intolerant individuals
- Soy protein—protein shake that is good for lactose-intolerant individuals
- Whey protein—protein shake derived from milk; can be used as a meal replacement and/or post-workout supplement; considered a fast digesting protein
- ZMA—great for muscle recovery, sleep agent, and keeping the body in an anabolic state

Supplements
Specific to Bulking Up vs. Toning Up

When building or toning muscle you want to make sure you are getting all of the vitamins you need. Consider taking a multi-vitamin. Also, for both processes you want to build lean muscle tissue. For this I recommend:

- Whey protein and casein protein help the body to rebuild the muscle tissues that were broken down during the workout. Take protein before and after your workouts as detailed in the protein section earlier in this chapter.
- Fish oils help the body to recover and help to keep the body in a muscle-building state. Take fish oils throughout the day as per the directions on the bottle.

Other supplements that I have found specifically helpful with the bulking up process:

- Creatine, in particular, helps with bulking up because it provides more energy for lifting heavier weights and helps you recover from short bursts of intense exercise. Take creatine about two hours before you lift weights.
- Glutamine is a great supplement for helping your body recover. Take glutamine before and after your workouts.

A Note on
Fat-Burning and/or Weight-Loss Pills

I get a lot of questions on the effectiveness of various fat-burning pills—whether they work and whether they are safe. A majority of fat-burning pills are mainly caffeine pills. Those that are can provide an energy boost if taken before your workout, but others have ingredients that can over-stimulate your heart rate, such as ephedra. Before ever taking any of these kinds of supplements, seriously consult with your physician.

My personal recommendation is to stay with more natural products and get your heart rate up the old fashioned way: good hard work!

Nutrition MYTHS

- Eating only low-fat foods will make you lose weight.
- Fat pills are all you need to look fit.
- You can't eat any carbs and lose weight.

Greg's Tips

- Eat lean proteins consisting of chicken, fish, lean beef, and turkey.

- Consume protein before eating carbohydrates to stabilize blood sugar levels. This is true for both snacks and meals. It is a great way to control blood sugar and appetite.

- Eat complex carbohydrates consisting of whole grains, oats, and vegetables.

- If possible, choose organic/natural foods.

- Eat healthy fats consisting of olive oil, nuts, fats from fish, and peanut butter.

- Drink water when you feel hungry to avoid eating when you are actually dehydrated.

- Drink at least eight 8-ounce glasses of water per day.

CHAPTER FOUR

Nutrition: Part II

*Changing the world around you begins
with changing you*

—Greg Marshall

Most people have a hard time with nutrition only because they aren't educated about what and when to eat. My goal is to help you understand the basics of nutrition and how to put meals together properly so that the fuel you consume properly meets your needs.

I want you to get so good at eating well that it will become a habit, and that you'll know how to have a balanced meal without even really thinking about it.

It is also necessary to understand the emotional and mental connection we all have with food. If you put the same work into your nutrition as you put into your workouts, I promise that you will see a drastic change in your progress.

It's always good to check with a doctor before you modify your diet.

Food and Emotion

Take a look at why you are eating, what you are eating, and when you are eating. How do you feel emotionally before you eat? What is your relationship with certain foods? Take time to analyze your food habits before you start to make changes in your lifestyle. If you don't understand your current lifestyle, the fitness and weight-loss strategies that you employ may not work, or the results won't last long-term. How you relate to food is just as important as what you eat.

One of my clients, Russell,[1] a healthy and fit executive who had exercised his whole life, struggled to reach his fitness goals, regardless of his dedication in the gym. Russ was a healthy eater: he always ate whole grains and fresh vegetables, he never smoked, and he didn't drink alcohol or even carbonated drinks. He shied away from anything resembling junk food. Yet, as he had approached his mid-forties, Russ's waistline continued to grow.

> *How you releate to food is just as important as what you eat.*

In exploring Russell's nutrition and food habits we identified two important issues. First, while he only ate healthy food, he ate a lot of it—often 3,000 calories a day for someone who should have been eating no more than 2,200. Second, he had a strong tendency, when stressed, to snack on (although healthy) high-calorie foods like almonds and pistachios. I had to explain to him that the only difference between a man who consumes 3,000 calories of good food each day and a man who consumes 3,000 calories of *junk* food, is that one guy feels a lot better than the other. However, both individuals will be overweight.

> *The only difference between a man who consumes 3,000 calories of good food each day and a man who consumes 3,000 calories of junk food, is that one guy feels a lot better than the other. Both are still overweight.*

Identifying triggers and causes for his weight gain helped Russ better control his eating habits.

For many people like Russ, eating can be a way of dealing with anxiety and stress. This isn't just a mental or emotional issue, it is a physiological one: food has the power to influence how we feel. Sugar increases serotonin levels, and serotonin makes us feel happy. When we are stressed, we want to feel happier, so we crave sugary foods to increase serotonin. This makes you much more likely to eat unhealthy foods, even though logically you know you shouldn't.

Keep in mind as you work to make changes in your diet that feeling stronger through eating well also increases serotonin. As you work to make yourself healthier, you will also be making yourself happier. You can create serotonin on your own without turning to the sugary food to do it for you.

Another client, Angela, told me the personal struggle she had with food addiction because of certain traumatic losses in her life. The easiest way for her to deal with the continuing feelings of guilt and anguish caused by these losses was to eat. She felt that food was the one thing she could count on to be there for her.

Because food was such an emotional hot button for her, no amount of diets or personal trainers could change Angela's weight. She had to work on solving the underlying issues that caused her overeating before she could make real changes to her eating habits.

It wasn't until Angela sought help from a licensed therapist that she began to see real progress with her fitness and weight goals.

Food Journal

Start a food journal. It's essential to be honest and use great detail. This can be as simple as keeping a notebook in your kitchen or workplace, or updating a note on your PDA, or entering thoughts on a calendar. There are also websites such as myfitnesspal. com, sparkpeople.com, and mypyramidtracker. com, as well as plenty of easy-to-use apps that allow you to track food intake. You can also make it a section in your fitness journal, which I introduced in "Getting Started."

> *Write how youe feel at the time of your meal. When you document your behavior in connection with your emotions, some suprising correlations can be found.*

Whatever software or system you use, just remember to find one that lets you track your emotional state at each meal. This can be an important component of whether a fitness program works or doesn't work. Also, choose software or apps that make sense to you and keep the process simple.

In your food journal, focus on more than just calories.

- Be sure to give the date and time of each meal.
- Write what you are eating *before* you eat it. Doing so will make you pay attention to what you are about to put into your body and will make you more conscious of your decisions, which usually leads to making healthier choices.
- Write how you are feeling at the time of your meal. When you document your behavior in connection with your emotions, some surprising correlations can be found.

Each morning, take a look at the previous day's entries. You may start to recognize trends. Is there a time of day that you find you are susceptible to overeating or making poor choices? Are you seeing certain emotions connected to eating certain foods? Watch for trends of negative feelings involved with eating or that cause cravings to eat. Ask yourself:

- Do I eat *because* I feel lonely, sad or depressed?
- Do I eat as self-punishment for not looking the way I think I am "supposed" to look?
- Do I tend to eat when I am bored?
- Do I eat to loneliness? And/or do I see meals as a social event?

Action Steps
to Replace Self-Sabotaging Behaviors

When you answer the above questions and see patterns of eating behaviors that work against you, cultivate replacement behaviors that directly address the root problem. For example, if you normally eat when you are lonely or bored, make a date with a friend to do something together that allows you to bond with the other person—like taking a walk. Try to plan activities in advance during the hours you tend to be most vulnerable to overeating. Some alternatives to eating that my clients have found helpful include:

- Learning how to play an instrument
- Joining a book club
- Learning a new skill
- Dating
- Spending time with your spouse or children
- Attending sporting events or concerts
- Practicing a hobby that requires your hands to stay clean or keep busy, such as sewing, crafting, or building models (or anything that keeps your hands too busy to put things in your mouth!)

Having a hobby can be an especially helpful diversion from mindless eating. It can often be done with family or friends—allowing time for socialization—but can also fill quiet hours for those of you who might otherwise find yourselves midnight snacking.

The objective is to find anything you can do to improve yourself and replace former self-sabotaging behaviors. Maybe you will even fall in love with your new endeavor and find another new passion!

Food Choices

Sustainability

Your nutrition choices should be healthy and sustainable. People make a mistake with their nutrition when they try to make radical changes with their diets. Instead, start with simple healthy choices. Substitute one healthy snack for a junk food snack and build from there. Remember that healthy foods fuel your body for exercise and keep you active so you feel better about yourself.

Focus on high quality nutrients for your system. The human body is like an expensive sports car. If you fuel it and maintain it correctly, it will perform well for years. If you neglect it and purchase poor fuel, the engine will give out. Our bodies truly are amazing things. They just need to be fueled with whole foods and the correct mixture of proteins, carbohydrates, fats, vitamins, and minerals.

Whole Foods and Your Body

The best way to get your body to respond to your workouts, as well as to assure you get the nutrition you need, is to eat foods that are in a whole state or in their natural form. The fewer ingredients that you see listed on the side of the packaging, the better the food is for you. Some nutritionists suggest you should never eat a packaged food with more than five ingredients. Work to minimize the number of the preservatives and foreign substances you put in your body.

Another good rule of thumb is, if you can't pronounce an ingredient, it's probably not good for you. Michael Pollan, the best-selling author of "In Defense of Food," says it this way: "Don't eat anything your great-grandmother wouldn't recognize as food."

On page 83 is a generic cookie nutrition label. You can see how many ingredients are listed. A basic cookie can be made with eggs, milk, flour, baking powder, salt, and brown sugar. The length of the ingredients list alone shows you that this item is probably an unhealthy food choice.

Preservatives and Processed Foods

A preservative is a foreign substance that companies add to food to extend shelf life. Preservatives make mass-produce foods possible. It has been said that we are an overfed but undernourished society—in my opinion that is because of the large amounts of processed foods we eat.

Processed foods add calories to your diet and don't fuel your body as efficiently as whole foods. After eating even a large meal of processed food, people feel full but often have low energy. This is because there are fewer nutrients in processed food. Low energy is your body's way of telling you that it lacks the key vitamins and minerals needed to keep it running efficiently.

Nutrition Facts

Serving Size 4 cookies (31g)
Servings Per Container about 9

Amount Per Serving

Calories 160   Calories from Fat 80

% **Daily Value***

Total Fat 9g	13%
Saturated Fat 6g	28%
Cholesterol 9mg	0%
Sodium 140mg	6%
Total Carbohydrate 20g	7%
Dietary Fiber 1g	5%
Sugars 11g	
Protein 1g	

Vitamin A 0%   •   Vitamin C 0%

Calcium 0%   •   Iron 2%

★ Percent Daily Values are based on a 2,000 calorie diet. Your daily values may be higher or lower depending on your calorie needs

Calories:	2,000	2,500
Total Fat	Less than	65g	80g
Sat Fat	Less than	20g	25g
Cholesterol	Less than	300mg	300mg
Sodium	Less than	2,400mg	2,400mg
Total Carbohydrate		300g	375g
Dietary Fiber		25g	30g

Calories per gram:
Fat 9 • Carbohydrate 4 • Protein 4

INGREDIENTS: ENRICHED FLOUR (WHEAT FLOUR, NIACIN, REDUCED IRON, THIAMINE MONO NITRATE, RIBOFLAVIN), SUGAR, VEGETABLE SHORTENING (CONTAINS ONE OR MORE OF THE FOLLOWING PARTIALLY HYDROGENATED OILS: PALM KERNEL, SOYBEAN, COTTONSEED, COCOA (PROCESSED WITH ALKALD, CARAMEL COLOR LEAVENING (SODIUM BI-CARBONATE, MONO CALCIUM PHOSPHATE, AMMONIUM BICARBONATE), HIGH FRUCTOSE CORN SYRUP, SALT, WHEY, SOY LECITHIN (EMULSIFIER), PEPPERMINT OIL, NATURAL AND ARTIFICIAL FLAVOR

Preservatives seem to be great for business but not for bodies. Most cereals, donuts, chips, and packaged meals are all full of preservatives. Most processed foods are in the middle of a grocery store, so as my friend, Tabitha, says, "shop around." That is, shop around the edges of the grocery store, where the whole food items are usually stocked: vegetables and fruit, dairy, and unadulterated meats.

Healthy Grocery Shopping

Grocery shopping must be done with intent. Prepare a list of healthy foods to purchase, don't browse. Most junk food choices are impulse purchases.

Half of the battle against eating junk food is fought at the grocery store. If you don't buy it, you don't bring it home and it isn't there to eat. It's okay to have a few junk foods in your house—everyone needs a treat now and again—but only buy them in small quantities. Don't keep too many high-calorie, low-nutrition snacks on hand. And don't use your kids as an excuse to buy cookies and candy. In fact, if you have kids, all the more reason *not* to buy junk food—they need healthy choices for snacking, too!

Never grocery shop when you have an empty stomach. When you're hungry you are more likely to buy foods that won't support your fitness goals.

When grocery shopping, visit stores that have a wide range of choices of organically grown fruits and vegetables, grass-fed beef, fresh fish, and chicken that haven't been treated with hormones. The labels on these foods will be marked to tell you if they are organic or not. Organic foods are not grown/raised/produced with chemicals, preservatives, or additives. Although it does cost a bit more to buy organic products, I can't think of a better investment than your food. You *are* what you eat.

Your grocery list should include fruits, vegetables, leans meats, whole grains and oats, water, olive oil, and some healthy snacks.

At the end of the chapter are two useful resources to help you with your grocery shopping, created by Laura Holtrop-Kohl MS, RD, CD, a dietician I have worked with from my local grocery store. I had her create a chart to help simplify the shopping and creation of good balanced meals—think of it as a Build a Balanced Meal Menu. The other document has reminders of how much and what to eat and gives some Health Lunch Ideas and Recipes.

Nutrition for Results

Calories

The chart on page 86 is from the National Institute of Health[2] and shows the estimated amount of calories you should eat each day to have the body function efficiently. It is based on gender, age, lifestyle, and activity levels.

Don't obsess about calories consumed versus calories burned, especially when you are at the beginning stages of your fitness journey. Just try to have an idea of your intake. If you are working out at the correct level of intensity (see "Resistance Training" and "Cardio" chapters), you should burn enough. Besides, if you compare

Gender	Age[1] (years)	Sedentary[2]	Moderately Active[3]	Active[4]
Child	2-3	1,000	1,000-1,400	1,000-1,400
Female	4-8	1,200	1,400-1,600	1,400-1,800
	9-13	1,600	1,600-2,000	1,800-2,200
	14-18	1,800	2,000	2,400
	19-30	2,000	2,000-2,200	2,400
	31-50	1,800	2,000	2,200
	51+	1,600	1,800	2,000-2,200
Male	4-8	1,400	1,400-1,600	1,600-2,000
	9-13	1,800	1,800-2,200	2,000-2,600
	14-18	2,200	2,400-2,800	2,800-3,200
	19-30	2,400	2,600-2,800	3,000
	31-50	2,200	2,400-2,600	2,800-3,000
	51+	2,000	2,200-2,400	2,400-2,800

1. These levels are based on Estimated Energy Requirements (EER) from the Institute of Medicine Dietary Reference Intakes macronutrients report, 2002, calculated by gender, age, and activity level for reference-sized individuals. "Reference size," as determined by IOM, is based on median height and weight for ages up to age 18 years of age and median height and weight for that height to give a BMI of 21.5 for adult females and 22.5 for adult males.

2. Sedentary means a lifestyle that includes only the light physical activity associated with typical day-to-day life.

3. Moderately active means a lifestyle that includes physical activity equivalent to walking about 1.5 to 3 miles per day at 3 to 4 miles per hour, in addition to the light physical activity associated with typical day-to-day life

4. Active means a lifestyle that includes physical activity equivalent to walking more than 3 miles per day at 3 to 4 miles per hour, in addition to the light physical activity associated with typical day-to-day life.

someone who eats 1200 calories of junk foods with someone who eats 2,000 calories of fish, nuts, and vegetables, who will be healthier and look better?

Remember, a healthy lifestyle is the goal and turning actions into a lifestyle takes practice.

Most diets that tell you to restrict calorie intake to ridiculously low levels are short-term programs and are not sustainable. Be practical and keep it simple. Track and measure everything that you eat and think long term.

Portion Size

The more you learn to control portion size the more results you will get. In the beginning it will feel overwhelming to pay attention to so many things at once, but when you practice the principles in this book they will become good habits to live by. Remember, a healthy lifestyle is the goal and turning actions into a lifestyle takes practice.

Train your body to get used to smaller more efficient meals. The portion sizes of proteins and carbs should each be no bigger than your fist. For example, a meal would include a fist size portion of chicken breast, a fist size portion of brown rice, and the rest of your plate should be filled with vegetables (and/or fruit).

Nutrition to Bulk Up vs. Nutrition to Tone Up

Nutrition to Bulk Up

If you are looking to increase muscle mass, or "bulk up," then you want to increase your calorie intake. It takes 3500 calories to gain a pound of weight. Simplified, you should increase your intake by 500 calories more per day than you normally eat. You must have a calorie surplus in order to increase your mass. If you normally eat 2000 calories per day, then eat 2500 calories per day. In my experience, increasing your calories too much too fast (such as increasing them by 700 or more per day) results in gaining excess body fat. When eating for bulk, be sure to eat healthy carbohydrates, proteins, fats, and vegetables/fruits in balanced meals.

I highly recommend eating one to one and a half grams of protein per pound of body weight per day when you are trying to bulk up. That is what works for me and for my clients.

Keep a daily food journal and specifically track grams of protein and caloric intake per day. Keep a very close eye on these numbers to make sure you are getting the necessary nutrients you need to "bulk up." And drink enough water so your body can

utilize all the nutrients you are eating.

Just because you gain a pound doesn't necessarily mean the pound is made of muscle. To make sure it is muscle you are amassing, you must be working out intensely with weights.

Nutrition to Tone Up

Usually a client who wants to tone also wants to lose weight. If that is the case, reduce your intake by 500 calories per day in order to lose a pound a week. For example, if you normally eat 2000 calories a day, then start eating 1500 calories per day. You don't want to reduce your overall caloric intake too much because you run the risk of losing energy as well muscle tissue. And believe me, you don't want to lose muscle, because muscle is what helps speed up your metabolism so you can burn more calories.

Also, you still need your body to feel it is getting enough calories—energy—to burn, especially when you are starting a new work out program, which is likely increasing your energy output. If you under-feed your body while over-extending energy output, your body may try to hang on to fat for storage.

Of course, those calories must come from high-quality foods so that your body is getting the nutrients necessary to increase your metabolism and allow you to exercise hard. Eat healthy carbohydrates, proteins, and fats in balanced meals.

Keep a daily food journal and specifically track grams of carbohydrates, protein, and calories. Be very detailed and accurate with everything you are eating to get the best results.

To aid toning, eat 1 gram of protein per pound of body weight each day. Focus on eating high-quality proteins (chicken, fish, and turkey; avoid red meat and pork) and high-quality fats such as olive oil, fish oil, nuts, and/or flaxseed oil. Somewhat minimize carbohydrate intake.

Based on your caloric needs (see chart above), you may want to replace some of your carbohydrate grams with grams of quality proteins and fats.

Drink enough water in order to utilize all the nutrients you are eating in your balanced meals.

Eat four to five times per day: three meals and one or two snacks per day. This will keep your metabolism at its peak and working to help you obtain your desired results.

How to Put Meals Together

By combining the right foods in each meal you can feel a difference in your moods and energy levels. Make sure there are the appropriate amounts of protein, carbohydrates, and fat in each meal. Even if you are making fairly nutritious, whole-food choices, you may not be giving yourself the balance of foods your body requires.

For example, whole-wheat toast and spreadable fruit (jelly without added sugar) are good choices as they are whole foods, but this isn't a complete meal. Both the bread and jelly are carbohydrates (natural sugars). Since there is no protein or fat in this meal, there is nothing to block the sugar spike (also known as an insulin spike) in your body. This means you will have a quick burst of energy followed by a severe drop in energy, often called a "crash." The crash is something you want to avoid if you are trying to live a healthy lifestyle. It's hard to have energy and motivation when you don't have the long-lasting fuel to back you up.

When you put your meals together, make sure that you have a high-quality fat, protein, and carb together. So if we add peanut butter (which has protein and fat in it) to the toast and jelly meal, the body will have short-term energy from the sugars and long-term energy from the protein and fat. This simple addition to the meal will help you have the energy to carry you through your activities until lunch.

If you feel like you are crashing during your day and unable to accomplish daily tasks, it could be because you aren't eating enough protein with your carbohydrates. For example, if you ate 30 grams of carbs in your breakfast and 10 grams of protein, and feel sluggish before lunch, change your breakfast intake to 20 grams of carbs and 20 grams of protein. Every person's body is different but these are some fundamentals. Track your food in your journal and test to see what works best for you.

Another common meal people enjoy is pasta, but most people eat pasta with tomato sauce and nothing else. This meal will give you the same problems that the toast and jelly did—even if you are choosing whole wheat pasta (which I would recommend). Add lean ground turkey or chicken breast with your pasta and sauce. Try to eat an almost equal amount of the turkey or chicken as pasta. Then add vegetables to the sauce or on the side. This will give you more flavor and provide the balance to complete the meal.

Speaking of vegetables, be aware that although potatoes and corn are plant-based, they are both considered carbohydrates due to their high starch content.

Three-Day Sample Menu

Remember that half the fight with food is planning ahead. In order to help you with that, here is a sample three-day menu, including snacks, so you can see how to put your meals together. Using a menu like this can help you begin to have a sense of how much and how often to eat, as well as what kinds of foods to pair together.

Think of this menu as a jumping off point. Adjust it based on your fitness goals (bulking or toning up) and the caloric intake chart provided earlier in this chapter.

Day 1

Meal 1:

- 2/3 cup oatmeal with frozen fruit
- 8 ounces water

Snack:

- Low-fat cheese stick
- 1 apple
- 8 ounces water

Meal 2:

- 1 pound baked or grilled chicken, sliced, with romaine lettuce
- 2 tablespoons light dressing (see "Nutrition: Part I, Sauces and Dressings" for ideas)
- 8 ounces water

Snack:

- Protein bar (less than 250 calories)

- 8 ounces water

Meal 3:

- 6 ounces tuna fish with two cups spinach
- 8 ounces water

Day 2

Meal 1:

- Protein shake mixed with 8 ounces water and 2/3 cup oatmeal

---

Snack:

- Low-sugar yogurt mixed with 1/2 cup granola
- 8 ounces water

Meal 2:

- Turkey sandwich using two slices of whole wheat bread with lettuce and mustard
- 8 ounces water

Snack:

- 1 handful of almonds or peanuts (unsalted)
- 8 ounces water

Meal 3:

- 4-ounce steak
- Romaine lettuce salad with oil and vinegar dressing
- 8 ounces water

Day 3

Meal 1:

- 3 slices turkey bacon on 1 slice whole wheat bread
- 8 ounces water

Snack:

- Protein bar (less than 250 calories)
- 8 ounces water

Meal 2:

- 1 cup whole wheat pasta with olive oil and 6 ounces of cooked, lean ground beef
- 8 ounces water

Snack:

- Whey protein smoothie mixed with 1 cup frozen fruit and 8–16 ounces water (based on how thick you want the smoothie to be.)

Meal 3:

- Lettuce salad with 1/4 cup sliced avocado
- 4 ounces grilled or baked chicken
- 8 ounces water

Other Meal-Building Resources

There are great websites (I recommend eatingwell.com, choose-myplate.gov, myfitnesspal.com, and bodybuilding.com) as well as cookbooks you can find for lean menu items. Just keep the basics from these nutrition chapters in mind as you are reading them and adjust as necessary to meet your own nutritional needs and goals.

You should also consider talking to your doctor and/or a licensed nutritionist if you need more direction or if you have any health issues to take into consideration.

Here are some other recipes I recommend, that you can find online:

www.eatingwell.com

- Baby Beet Greens with Spicy Mediterranean Vinaigrette
- Beer-Battered Fish Tacos with Tomato and Avocado Salsa
- Chicken and Fruit Salad
- Chili-rubbed Steaks and Pan Salsa
- Rainbow Chopped Salad
- Seared Steak Salad with Edamame and Cilantro
- Shrimp Cobb Salad
- Southwestern Beef and Bean Burger Wraps

Greg's Tips

- Eat slowly and chew your food completely. This helps digestion. It also takes time for the message "I'm full" to travel from the stomach to the brain.

- Eat small meals and snacks throughout the day to curb your appetite and increase your energy.

- Grocery shop after a meal, never when you are hungry. And "shop around" the edges of the store where the whole foods tend to be offered.

- If possible, choose organic/natural foods.

- Find healthy foods you enjoy and get creative with how you prepare them.

- Buy a healthy recipe book to give you ideas on how to add variety to your meals.

- Do not mistake nutrition for a "diet," which has a negative connotation.

- Each meal should have a protein and a carbohydrate together to stabilize blood sugar.

Choose One or More from Each Column to Build a Better Meal

Protein	Grains	Vegetables	Fruit	Dairy
Hummus	Quick Barley	Avocado	Apple	Blue Cheese
Kidney Beans	Low Sugar Granola	Bell Pepper	Apricot	Cottage Cheese
Black Beans	Instant Oatmeal	Broccoli	Banana	Feta
Garbanzo Beans	Popcorn	Cabbage	Blackberries	Fortified Soy Milk
Pinto Beans	Quinoa	Carrot	Blueberries	Frozen Yogurt
Split Peas	Whole Grain Bulgur Wheat	Cauliflower	Cantaloupe	Goat Cheese
Refried Beans	Whole Grain Cereal	Celery	Cherries	Light Spreadable Cheese
Lentils	Whole Grain Corn Bread	Corn	Clementine	Milk
Nuts	Whole Grain Corn Chips	Cucumber	Dried Fruit	Pudding (made with milk)
Peanut Butter	Whole Grain Crackers	Edamame	Fruit Juice	Reduced Fat Cream Cheese
Almond Butter	Whole Grain Pita Bread	Jicama	Grapes	Ricotta
Sunflower Seeds	Whole Grain Sandwich Bread	Lentils	Honeydew Melon	String Cheese

Protein	Grains	Vegetables	Fruit	Dairy
Pumpkin Seeds	Whole Grain Tortilla	Lettuce	Kiwi	Vegetable Dip Made with Low-Fat Yogurt
Pine Nuts	Whole Grain Waffle	Onions	Mango	Yogurt
Texturized Vegetable Protein	Whole Wheat Bagel	Peas	Orange	
Tempeh	Whole Wheat Couscous	Potato	Papaya	
Tofu	Whole Wheat English Muffin	Pumpkin	Peach	
Egg	Whole Wheat Hamburger Bun	Radishes	Pears	
Chicken Breast	Whole Wheat Pasta	Spinach	Pineapple	
Turkey Brest	Whole Wheat Pizza Crust	Sugar Snap Peas	Raspberries	
Tuna		Tomato	Strawberries	
Salmon		Vegetable Juice	Watermelon	
Lean Pork		Winter Squash		
Lean Beef		Zucchini		

Fresh and Healthy
Brown Bag Lunch Workshop

Packed lunches are a great way to control what you're eating. However, many of us get stuck in the "ham sandwich, apple, and chips" rut. So, how do we escape the rut and make lunches from home both enjoyable and nutritious? Let's start with the nutrition:

What goes into a healthy lunch?

When creating a lunch, aim for 1/4 of your lunch coming from protein, 1/4 from grains, and 1/2 coming from fruits and vegetables. Then add one serving of dairy. Eating a lunch proportioned this way will help you to meet your body's nutrition needs for the day. The exact amount on your plate will vary depending on your age, gender, and calorie needs.

Protein

Protein is needed by your body to build and repair itself, to fight infections and to help your body to regulate its many functions. Your first thought when protein is mentioned may be proteins such as meat, poultry, and fish, but eggs, dairy products, nuts, seeds, beans, or tofu are excellent options as well. When you choose meat or poultry as your protein source, be sure to choose lean sources. For an adult consuming 2,000 calories per day about 5.5 ounces of protein foods are needed in a day, so 2–3 ounces of protein is a good amount to plan for lunch.

An Ounce of Protein is:

- 1 ounce fish, meat or poultry
- 1 egg
- 1/2 ounce nuts or seeds
- 1 tablespoon nut butter
- 1/4 cup beans
- 2 tablespoons hummus
- 1/4 cup (2 ounces) tofu

Grains

Grains provide carbohydrates that your body needs for energy, as well as important vitamins and minerals. At least half of your grains each day should be whole grains; not only do whole grains provide fiber that promotes digestive health, but they may reduce your risk of heart disease, cancer, and diabetes. For an adult consuming 2,000 calories per day, 6 ounces of grains are needed in a day, so aim for 2 ounces of grains at lunch.

An Ounce of Grains is:

- 1 slice bread
- 1/2 large pita bread
- 3 cups popped popcorn
- 1 ounce whole grain crackers
- 1/2 cup cooked rice or pasta
- 1 small (6-inch diameter) tortilla
- 1 piece of thin crust medium pizza
- 1/2 piece of thick crust medium pizza

Fruits and Vegetables

Fruits and vegetables provide important vitamins and minerals as well as fiber for digestive health and carbohydrates for energy. Eating a variety of fruits and vegetables may reduce your risk of heart disease, some types of cancer, and diabetes. For an adult consuming 2,000 calories per day, 2 cups of fruit and 2 1/2 cups of vegetables are needed. As most people don't eat vegetables at breakfast, it is important that you choose to add vegetables to your lunch to ensure that you eat enough to meet your needs for the day.

A Cup of Vegetables or Fruit is:

- 1 cup of raw or cooked vegetables or fruit
- 1 cup cooked beans, lentils, or split peas
- 1 small or 1/2 large piece of fruit
- 1 large bell pepper, tomato, or ear of corn
- 1 medium potato
- 1/2 cup dried fruit
- 1 cup of 100% fruit or vegetable juice
- 2 cups raw, leafy greens (1 cup cooked)
- 3 cups tomato soup

Dairy

Dairy products are great sources of calcium and phosphorus which are essential in building and maintaining healthy bones and teeth. They also provide carbohydrates for energy, and potassium, which helps maintain healthy blood pressure. Milk and some yogurts have vitamin D added, which helps your body to absorb the calcium and phosphorus. Choose low- or non-fat dairy sources more often. For those who do not consume dairy, calcium and vitamin D fortified non-dairy options, such as soy milk, are a good option. Children 9 years or older and all adults should consume three servings of dairy per day. Aim for at least one serving of dairy at lunch.

A Serving of Dairy is:

- 1 cup milk or yogurt
- 1 cup calcium-fortified soy milk
- 1 1/2 ounces natural cheese
- 1/3 cup shredded natural cheese
- 2 ounces processed cheese
- 1/2 cup ricotta cheese
- 2 cups cottage cheese
- 1 cup frozen yogurt
- 1 1/2 cups ice cream
- 1 cup pudding (made with milk)

Equipment

The next step in planning your lunch is to consider what equipment you have available to you. This will help you to decide what types of food you can safely bring with you. Do you have a refrigerator available or will you be using an insulated lunch bag with a cold pack? Do you have an insulated food jar to keep foods hot or do you have a microwave to heat foods? What other equipment do you have available?

Putting It All Together

Now that you know how many servings of different types of foods you should have, and have considered what equipment you have available to you, it is time to plan some imaginative and delicious lunches.

Sample Cold Lunch Menus

- Vegetarian Pita Sandwich
  and 1/2 cup ricotta mixed with 1/2 cup blackberries.

  The Sandwich is made with 1 whole grain pita pocket, 1/4 cup hummus, 1 cup spinach and 1/2 cup mixed vegetables (sliced cucumber, grated carrot and diced tomato are great for this) drizzled with 2 tablespoons tzaziki sauce.

- Spring Salad
  served with a Whole Grain Roll

  Spring Salad is made with 2 cups mixed baby lettuces, 1/2 cup berries, 1 1/2 ounces crumbled feta cheese, 1 ounce of walnuts (about 14 halves) with a lite raspberry dressing such as Annie's Lite Raspberry Vinaigrette or Newman's Own Raspberry & Walnut Dressing.

- Chicken, Rice and Black Bean Salad
  served with 1 cup pineapple chunks

  Salad is made by tossing together 1/2 cup cold brown rice, 1/2 cup cold shredded chicken breast, 1/2 cup black beans, 1 chopped Roma tomato, 1 sliced green onion, 1 teaspoon minced cilantro, 1/3 cup shredded low-fat cheese. Take the dressing (made with 1 tablespoon white wine vinegar, 1 tablespoon olive oil, 1/2 teaspoon minced jalapeno or 1/8 teaspoon chipotle powder, a pinch of cumin and a dash of salt and pepper) separately in a small container and toss with the salad at lunch-time a dressing.

- Tabbouleh Salad
  served with 1/2 turkey, Gouda and apple sandwich

  Tabbouleh Salad is made by combining 1/2 cup cooked whole grain bulgur wheat, 1/2 cup chopped cucumber, 1/2 cup chopped tomato, 1 tablespoon chopped mint, 2 tablespoons chopped parsley, 1 tablespoon lemon juice, 1 teaspoon olive oil, and a pinch of cumin. The sandwich is made with 2 ounces of reduced sodium turkey breast, 1 slice of gouda cheese, 1/2 small apple, and 1 teaspoon honey mustard on 1 slice whole grain bread (cut in half).

- Tuscan Tuna Salad
  served with 2 ounces whole grain crackers and 1 container yogurt mixed with 1/2 cup cut fruit

  Tuscan Tuna Salad is made with 1 3-ounce can chunk light tuna in water (drained), 1/2 cup low-sodium cannellini beans, 1/2 cup halved cherry tomatoes, 1 tablespoon minced shallot, 1 tablespoon parsley, 1 teaspoon lemon juice, and 1 teaspoon olive oil.

Sample Hot Lunch Menus

- Barbecue Chicken Sandwich
  served with coleslaw and Watermelon Salad.

  Heat 1/2 cup shredded chicken breast with 2 tablespoons of your favorite barbecue sauce and serve on a whole-wheat hamburger bun. Make coleslaw with 1 cup of precut coleslaw blend and 2 tablespoons vinaigrette such as Litehouse Fuji Apple Vinaigrette. Watermelon Salad is made with 1 cup watermelon chunks, 1 cup non-fat plain Greek yogurt, 1 tablespoon minced mint, and 1 tablespoon lime juice.

- Hearty Tomato Soup, "grilled" cheese sandwich, and 3 fresh clementines.

  Make Hearty Tomato Soup by pureeing 1/2 cup low-sodium great northern beans into 1 can no-sodium added tomato soup (taste and add a dash of salt if needed); heat and eat. Pack 2 slices toasted whole grain bread and 1 1/2 ounces cheddar cheese; using a microwave heat on high for about 30 seconds for a "grilled" cheese sandwich.

- Bean Burrito,
  1/2 cup tropical mixed fruit (mango, pineapple, and papaya),
  1/2 cup Harmons Corn and Black Bean Salad.

  To make burrito, spread 1/2 cup low-sodium refried beans and 1/3 cup shredded cheese on a large whole-wheat tortilla; heat in microwave. Add 2 tablespoons salsa and 1/2 cup vegetables (such as romaine lettuce, diced tomato, and onion), wrap and enjoy.

- Chicken Pasta
  with Marinara Sauce, mini-sweet peppers with goat cheese, and a peach.

  Cook 2 ounces whole wheat pasta. When cooked toss with 1/2 cup low-sodium marinara sauce such as Dave's Gourmet Spicy Heirloom Marinara and 1/2 cup pre-cooked chicken breast strips. Cut 2 mini sweet peppers in half and stuff with 1 1/2 ounces of your favorite goat cheese.

CHAPTER FIVE

Resistance Training

Your results are past your comfort zone.

- G.M.

Why Resistance Training Is Necessary and How to do It

Resistance training, strength training, and weight-lifting training are synonymous terms. It is the use of weights or any kind of resistance to break down the muscle fibers so that they can be built back up in better form. The tools used in resistance training are dumbbells, barbells, kettle bells, strength-training machines, and your own body weight.

Resistance training is not just something bodybuilders do. Many people—especially women—avoid using weights because they think it will make them overly muscular. This is one of the biggest misconceptions that people have. If you are looking to add muscle mass to your body, you must have a nutrition plan to support that goal. Simply using strength-training exercises won't create large muscles. You must *try* to bulk up if you are going to get "bulky."

What strength training through weight resistance does on its own is decrease body fat and tone your muscles. The process makes the muscle fibers more efficient at burning calories and the new muscle that you add to your body—replacing fat—will enhance your metabolism, making long-term results more attainable. If you want to continuously burn calories while you are awake, asleep, or working out, you *must* build muscle.

Another reason some women are afraid to use weights is because they see increases on the scale early on during the process. This is because some muscle will be built *before* the fat is initially burned. Stick with the resistance training and the weight will come off and lean muscle will take its place.

I am often asked how many **sets** (a group of repetitions) and **repetitions** (known as "reps": the number of times you do an exercise without stopping) should be done for the perfect workout. There is no magic number. You should be continuously striving to increase the level of resistance to help change your body. This is a marathon, not a sprint. Different bodies respond differently, so track your workouts in a fitness journal from your first day and monitor the changes.

Note: Don't simply mimic workout plans from fitness models. Doing their programs could possibly injure you. It is hard to get results when you have to start and stop because of injuries. Check with your doctor or consult with a personal trainer and/or nutritionist before beginning any workout program. Then start carefully and slowly using the recommendations in this book.

Keeps tabs on how you feel and start out easy. There is a difference between being sore and being injured. Unless you are injured, you should still be mobile. If you are feeling tightness, you are sore; if you are experiencing sharp pain, this indicates a possible injury. If the pain lasts more than three or four days and still feels severe you should see a doctor.

All major resistance exercises are shown in the "Exercise Glossary" at the end of this book.

Hypertrophy

Don't feel intimidated by the scientific term. **Hypertrophy** (pronounced /hiy-PUR-truh-fee/) is just a fancy way of saying "building muscle."

Now, before some of you get scared, building muscle is *not* the same as bodybuilding. Although, in my opinion, bodybuilders aren't just 300-pound muscle men or people who can lift cars with their chins. A bodybuilder can be a 130-pound woman who is toning up her body to burn more calories. We can *all* be bodybuilders; the question is *how* we build, and how *much* we build our bodies.

Both men and women can benefit from adding muscle mass, so don't steer away from these goals if you are aiming to lose weight and tone up. You have control of how much muscle mass you want to add by the combination of your nutrition, resistance routine, and cardio (see "Bulking Up vs. Toning Up" sections in this and related chapters).

Back to hypertrophy. The best way to tell if you are hitting a state of hypertrophy is if you are gaining more muscle tissue. The optimal way to track your progress and see how much muscle you have and are gaining is through a body fat analysis (see "Getting Started"). But often you can simply see the results in the mirror given a month or so of healthy eating, proper caloric intake, and good, consistent resistance training.

Can You Resistance Train Your Full Body Every Day?

My philosophy on training is that there is no such thing as a "perfect" system. I don't believe any training philosophy that says there is only one way to achieve your goals. Every person's body is different and will respond to different methods of training. But there are ways to personalize your training and there are certain methods that seem to help most, as well as some new ideas about how to go about the process.

The key to getting your own best results is by understanding the different tools that you have available and how certain exercises will help you meet certain goals. By having this knowledge, you can test out and track different workouts and training methods that work for you.

In the past it was believed that resistance training your full body every day was "overtraining." Many people thought that the body needed rest days. Actually, in my experience, and according to some studies going on now, not only is it *possible* to train your full body five days a week, but doing so increases results and can help reduce injuries—as long as you follow some basic guidelines.

The trick to full-body training is that while you may exercise all major muscle groups, you focus the intensity and most of the repetitions on just one or two muscle groups per day, and alternate the muscle groups that do the bulk of the work every other day.

The decision to resistance train your full body at every workout session depends on the results you are striving to achieve, and you must consider the load, resistance, and sequence of exercises.[1]

The **load** refers to the amount of resistance that you give your muscles in a given day. You can't do the same load on the same muscle every day using drop sets (that is, lifting until muscle failure —described in detail later in this chapter). This *will* over train your muscles and increase your chances of injury.

The level of **resistance** your muscles experience should change daily by choosing different muscle groups to train. For example, if you are training your chest each day, then instead of doing a flat bench press daily, choose an incline bench press to work out your upper chest on alternate days. This will at least give you an opportunity to focus on a different part of that muscle group, while not overtraining one specific area.

Large muscle groups:

- Arms (biceps, triceps)

- Shoulders

- Chest

- Back

- Legs (hamstrings, quadriceps, calves)

The **sequences** of exercises you perform should focus on different parts of the body on alternating days. So, if you are going to perform six different exercises and you are emphasizing your workout on chest muscles, then four of the exercises would be for the chest and two would be for another part of the body, like the legs. On the following day, switch your emphasis.

Another example: if you do most of your exercises on the upper half of your body during one day's workout, then the next day do more lower body exercises while still working out your upper body. This will take some stress off of certain muscle groups every day, while still being able to train them all to get full-body results.

Note: A good way to switch it up every other week or so would be to just change the organization of the workout. So if you did each exercise for two sets before, you could do each exercise for one set, going through all the exercises, then do another set for each exercise.

Example of Full-Body Training

Upper Body Day

1. Warm-Up activities, 10 minutes

    (Choose one): stationary bike, elliptical, treadmill, jog outside, walk, walking lunges, jumping jacks, vibration platform

2. Resistance

Large Muscle Group:
- Bench press, 2—3 sets of 10—12 reps
- Back rows, 2—3 sets of 10—12 reps
- Shoulder press, 2—3 sets of 10—12 reps

Small Muscle Group:
- Bicep curl, 2—3 sets of 10—12 reps
- Triceps push-down, 2—3 sets of 10—12 reps

3. Cardio: Treadmill, run 20 minutes

4. Cool Down: flexibility and stretching exercises

Lower Body Day

1. Warm Up activities, 10 minutes

   (Choose one): stationary bike, elliptical, treadmill, jog outside, walk, walking lunges, jumping jacks, vibration platform

2. Cardio: Stationary bike, 20 minutes

3. Resistance:

   Large Muscle Group:
   - Squats, 2—3 sets of 10—12 reps
   - Lunges, 2—3 sets of 10—12 reps
   - Step-ups, 2—3 sets of 10—12 reps

   Small Muscle Group
   - Calf Raises 2—3 sets of 10—12 reps

4. Cardio: Treadmill, run 20 minutes

5. Cool Down: flexibility and stretching exercises

Focus on Your Form

When you are resistance training, your form is going to dictate how well your body responds to the exercise program. Form is often a confusing concept for novice exercisers. Having never lifted weights before, they are, for the most part, guessing. Let's take the guesswork out of the equation.

First, every time you lift weights your core should be tight. What this means is that you should be tightening, or pulling in, your abdominal muscles to make sure that you are stabilizing your body. This will help to keep your body in the correct position and aligned properly so that you don't injure yourself.

Next, when you are positioning your body, it should be aligned naturally. Your feet should face forward and not point in or out. You should be in an athletic stance: feet shoulder-width to slightly-wider-than-shoulder-width apart. With your core tightened, your back should be straight at all times (no arching).

Anytime you do a squat, lunge, or any leg movement, your knees should bend no further than lining up with your toes. Also, never "lock out" (hyper-extend) any of your joints when performing a movement pattern. For example, if you are doing a bicep curl, never allow your elbow to completely extend to where your arm is straight.

You should never feel like you are in an awkward position and none of your joints should feel like they are pinching or getting aggravated by the movements. If you feel pain in any of your joints when you are resistance training, immediately correct your form. If your form is good and you still feel pain, then stop. See a physician before you continue training.

When using weights, repetitions should be controlled. It typically takes anywhere from three to five seconds total to complete one repetition. For example, if you are going to perform one rep of a bicep curl, then take three to five seconds to start in the extension position, come up to the fully flexed position, and return back to the appropriate extension position. (See "Exercise Glossary" for pictures of correct form.)

Exhale as the muscle contracts and inhale as the muscle releases with each repetition, and put 100 percent of your focus and energy on feeling your muscles contract and relax through every rep.

Paying close attention to your form will help you avoid injury and help you obtain the best results possible.

Is it Working?

How do you know that you are doing the exercise correctly? The muscles you are training should feel the burn but you shouldn't experience any joint pain. You should feel extra blood pumping into your muscles, and it will give you a feeling that your muscles are bigger than their normal state. For people trying to lose weight, this is sometimes scary as they think that the exercises are making them bulky. This is not the case. Your nutrition and caloric intake are what make the difference in how your muscles respond after you train (see chapters on nutrition and "Putting it Together").

If you are not feeling a burn and are completing your allotted reps easily, then it is time to increase the weight and/or the number of reps.

Remember, as I discussed in reference to plateaus in previous chapters, if you are not continuously pushing yourself in your workouts, you will get stuck. Plateaus are probably going to occur no matter what, but don't help them by not pushing yourself a little every day.

Muscular Imbalance

Muscular imbalance is one of the leading causes of injury. The imbalances cause one side of the body to dominate the other side, putting additional stress on the weaker side and leading to a pull, strain, or tear.

An example of this is the hamstring pull, the most common injury that we hear about in sports. We are all, for the most part, quadriceps (front-of-thighs) dominant. Quadriceps dominant refers to our tendency to do everything in forward motion. We walk forward, we run forward, we tend to resistance train the muscles we can see: like, obviously, the quadriceps.

This causes our quadriceps to be stronger than our hamstrings (back and inner thigh), so when there is an intense burst of speed or sprint, the hamstring is not prepared to handle the intensity. Because of imbalance, the hamstring is easily injured.

The best way to avoid muscular imbalance is to always do the same amount of sets, reps, and intensity for the muscles on the front of your body as the back of your body. Let me be clear: the weight level doesn't need to be equal, But the level of effort does.

The best way to avoid muscular imbalance is to always do the same amount of sets, reps, and intensity for the muscles on the front of your body as the back of your body. Let me be clear: "the same intensity" doesn't mean using the same weight or resistance level for, say, your hamstrings as your quads. It is, rather, matching the level of *effort* you are putting into an exercise. For example, if your hamstring was injured, lighter amounts of weights or a lower resistance level will challenge it. Then make sure that you use whatever weight level is necessary to challenge your quads. The weight level doesn't need to be equal. But the level of effort does.

Common muscle imbalances:

- performing abdominal crunches, without working out the lower back

- performing bench press for the chest, without back rows for the back

- performing leg curls for the quads, without leg extensions for the hamstrings

You don't necessarily have to do the back-body work the same day as the front-body work. But if you don't, try to do them on consecutive days. Track your workouts to make sure you are training both the front and back of the body equally throughout the week (just as you want to equally train the left and right sides of your body).

If you are already in a workout program, try to focus your next three to four days of workouts on your backside muscles, such as upper back, lower back, hamstrings, and triceps.

Bulking Up vs. Toning Up

Here it is, this is what most of you are looking to specifically understand: the differences between increasing muscle mass and build—or, as we commonly call it, **bulking up**—and slimming or refining the body: **toning up**. Generally speaking, men are focusing on the former and women on the latter, but that's not always the case, so I'll keep gender references neutral.

Resistance Training to Bulk Up

In order to increase muscle mass you want to focus your workouts on compound exercises such as the bench press and squat. When done correctly and with enough weight, compound exercises will stimulate the muscles to grow—much more so than doing isolation exercises on cable press machines and stationary machines.

If your goal is to bulk up, lift the heaviest weights you can for sets of five to eight reps. This assumes that you already have a workout in place. If you don't, start the first few weeks with light weights and slowly work your way up to the heavy ones.

The key is to make sure you are pushing yourself to your max and lifting the heaviest weights possible. Lift the weights in a controlled fashion without arching your back or locking, or hyper-extending your knees or elbows. Good form is always of utmost importance to getting the most out of your workout and preventing injury.

Also make sure that you are paying close attention to how your muscles feel and that you focus your effort on the desired muscle group. For example, when doing the bench press, pay attention that the chest muscles are doing the brunt of the work. I often notice clients use their shoulders to do the work, rather than their chest.

Focus 100 percent of your energy on making the muscle you are trying to work do all of the exercise. At the point of contraction be sure you are breathing out and at the point of lengthening, breathe in. For example, when you do a bench press, exhale as you push the weight up and inhale as you are bring the bar down towards your body. This should be a natural breathing pattern.

Earlier in this chapter I stated that you could work out your full body every day. But if your goal is to bulk up, you need to really push your muscles as far as they can go. So to bulk, it is key that each workout day uses *only* one or two large muscle groups (such as chest and triceps on one day, back and biceps on the next) at high intensity, while allowing the other muscle groups to recover until the alternate day.

For a four-day workout program, separate into the following muscle groups:

- Chest and triceps

- Back and biceps

- Shoulders

- Legs (hamstrings, quadriceps, calves)

Resistance Training to Tone Up

Many times when people want to tone up, they avoid resistance training. Don't. Resistance training is what makes muscles lean.

Toning up usually means losing fat and increasing lean muscle. This means a fair amount of cardio work needs to be done (see "Cardio"), but you still want to build muscle to increase your metabolism.

It is a myth that using high numbers of repetitions with weights that don't challenge your muscles at all will create definition. It just won't. If I lifted a pen for 1,000 reps every day it wouldn't create lean muscle tissue. You should always be challenging the muscle. Muscles have to be challenged to become toned.

Many times when people want to tone up, they avoid resistance training. Don't. Resistance training is what makes muscles lean.

For those who want to tone but who don't necessarily want to lose weight, the best balance is twenty minutes of cardio and forty minutes of resistance training.

Whether you need the weight loss, just the toning, or both, aim for eventually exercising five to six days per week for best results. For the highest calorie burn, focus your resistance training on

> *Muscles have to be challenged to become toned.*

one or two muscle groups as part of full-body workouts.

Focus on exercises that work large muscle groups such as squats, bench presses, deadlifts, shoulder presses, and back rows. Choose three or four resistance exercises. Do two or three sets of 10 to 15 reps for each exercise. Perform the exercises with high intensity, and rest very minimally (if at all) between sets. The goal is to perform 30- to 60-minute workouts with as little rest as possible. This will keep your body in a calorie-burning mode.

If you are a beginner, you can use cable and stationary machines, but use those that work large muscle groups like the chest press machine or lat pull-down machine. Avoid those that you may read about in workout and health magazines that isolate a single muscle (called *isolations*), such as the seated calf-raise or the forearm curl machines. You need to build up some good strength across the large muscle groups before isolating the small muscles. As I like to say, you want to build a strong foundation before you put on the roof!

Take anywhere between a month to two months of consistent exercise working out large muscle groups, making sure you are confident that your form and techniques are correct, before incorporating isolations into your routine.

As you get stronger, increase the weights and complexity of exercises.

Abdominals

Almost anyone that is working out wants the stomach area defined and toned. Strong abs can be a kind of a trophy of fitness. Unfortunately, most people believe that doing hundreds of abdominal exercises will get them results, but that isn't really the most effective approach. While exercises help build up the muscle, the main thing most people need to do is reduce body fat percentage in order to reveal the muscle underneath.

When resistance training, you should be paying close attention to keeping your core tight so that your abdominals are getting a workout from *all* of your movement patterns—not just the abs-focused exercises like crunches.

When doing abdominal exercises, be sure that you are flexing your abdominals during *the entire crunch* to ensure that the abs are getting the stimulation that they need. That's right. Keep your stomach flexed tightly while you are moving forward *and* while you are moving backward during the crunch. Also, be sure to breathe in and out with the movements, breathing out at the point of muscle contraction.

Key Abdominal Exercises: These are the most challenging abdominal exercises and they mostly use your own body weight, which helps to strengthen the muscles that can help you in day-to-day activities.

- Bosu ball crunch
- Hanging leg raise
- Decline abs crunch

- Medicine ball crunch

- Physioball crunch

- Reverse crunch

- Roman chair lift

Sets and Lifts

There has been quite a debate about how many sets or repetitions a person should do in order to get any given desired outcome, be it gaining muscle, toning, or losing fat. I don't believe there is any magic bullet for working out, so based on your abilities, try these rep techniques and see what works for you.

- To Increase Strength and Power: one to three repetitions with a minute to two minutes rest in between sets.

- To Promote Hypertrophy (Muscle Growth): eight to fifteen repetitions with a minute rest or less in between sets.

- To Increase Muscular Endurance: fifteen repetitions or higher with less than thirty seconds rest in between sets.

Types of Sets

Straight Set

A straight set is doing repetitions of an exercise followed by a rest period of anywhere from thirty seconds to three minutes before starting the set again. The most popular straight set recommended is three sets of ten repetitions of the same exercise. An example would be doing a set of squats for ten repetitions and then resting for a minute and performing another set of ten. Rest, repeat. A straight set is a great place for a fitness beginner to start.

Super Set

A super set is performing two different exercises in a row without a rest. For example, doing a squat for ten reps followed immediately by a walking lunge for ten reps without resting in between. Super sets are great to put your body in a state of hypertrophy.

There are sub-types of super sets such as **protagonist super sets,** where you perform two exercises with no rest in between for the same muscle group (for example, the chest). There are also **antagonist super sets,** where you perform two different exercises for opposing muscle groups. For example, the bench press for the chest followed by the seated row for the back (these are great for maintaining body muscle balance).

Tri-Set

A tri-set is a group of three exercises that are performed in sequence with no rest in between. Tri-sets are an effective way to increase the intensity of your workout and also allow you to get in a state of hypertrophy. For example, a chest tri-set would include performing a bench press, followed by a push-up, followed by a dumbbell fly without resting. This is a technique that is used by both bodybuilders and fitness models.

Drop Set

A drop set is continuously performing an exercise until you reach muscle failure (the inability to do any more repetitions at that weight), followed by decreasing the resistance weight by five or ten pounds and repeating the cycle until you reach absolute muscle failure.

For example, you would perform a machine bench press, beginning at a challenging—but not extremely difficult—weight for you. For the purpose of this example, let's say 100 pounds. Continue repetitions until you are unable to push the machine up again, then decrease the weight to 90 pounds and continue with the exercise until it again becomes too difficult. Drop the weight to 80 pounds and continue, etc.

This is a very intense resistance training technique, so I recommend performing drop sets on machines as they are safer for this activity than free weights.

This set is intense, but beginners can do it because the intensity is based on a weight load or resistance level that is challenging but not extremely difficult *for you.*

Giant Set

A giant set is four or more exercises performed in sequence with less than sixty seconds rest in between. This is a very intense resistance-lifting technique and would be considered advanced. Because of its intensity, this is a set-lift technique that you would slowly work up to. I don't recommend it for beginners.

For example, a giant set for the back muscles would include a seated row, followed by a lateral pull-down, deadlift, and a dumbbell row. This is also a great technique to hit muscle hypertrophy.

Types of Lifts

You always want to start with exercising large muscle groups before exercising a single muscle. Large muscle groups are worked by compound lifts. Single muscles are worked using isolation lifts.

Compound Lifts

Compound exercises are historically the most well-known because they require so much energy to perform and are typically the foundation of a resistance-training program. These exercises are considered the best for overall body strength, increased muscle mass, and for balancing out the body.

However, if you have had a back or large-joint injury, I don't recommend starting with compound lifts. The movements put so much stress on the joints that if your body is not prepared for the movements, you can seriously injure yourself.

Examples of Compound Lifts:

- Bench press
- Deadlift
- Lunge
- Pull-up
- Push-up
- Shoulder press (also known as *military press*)
- Squat and jump squat
- Step-up

Isolation Lifts

Isolation exercises are movement patterns that only require one muscle. These exercises are great for helping to rehabilitate an injury, build a specific muscle group for bodybuilding purposes, or to even out muscular imbalances.

Examples of Isolation Lifts:

- Abdominal machines
- Bicep curl
- Bicep machines
- Cable curl
- Calf machines
- Dumbbell curl

- Forearm/wrist curls

- Front raise

- Lateral raise

- Leg curl

- Leg extension

- Triceps machines

- Triceps push-down

Resistance Training and Weight-lifting Tools

There are several tools that you can use in order to do resistance training. They include the dumbbell, barbell, kettle bell, cable machines, your own body weight, water, and anything else that gives resistance to a movement pattern that you perform. Each tool stimulates your muscles somewhat differently, but all are versatile and can be used to achieve your goals.

Which type of resistance training you choose depends on how you want to accomplish the goal of breaking down your muscles so that you can build them back up when you rest and eat a nutritious diet. My suggestion is to first use what is available to you, and then switch it up every couple of weeks so that your whole body can get a feel for different angles and movements. The more variety you add to your workouts, the better results you will get.

Dumbbells

Dumbbells are great if you want to activate your core and correct muscle imbalances. The benefits of using dumbbells include making you use both the front and back of your body and helping to stimulate your stabilizer muscles (abs and lower back).

Dumbbells offer a variety of exercises for all muscle groups. If you're new to using dumbbells, be sure to start with light weights and progressively increase the weight each week. I typically suggest starting with the lightest weight possible and practicing the movements with careful attention to the correct form until you can perform at least a week's worth of workouts with good form and technique, before moving on to heavier weights.

If your body is hurting in any way when performing the exercises, stop and check your form. The movement should feel natural. If it does not, you are likely putting your body at risk for injury. Pay close attention.

When training with dumbbells, you will typically need a flat bench or an adjustable bench in order to perform movement patterns for your chest, back, shoulders, and legs. A bench can greatly enhance the benefits of dumbbells because of the versatility it offers. Also consider investing in a rubber mat, so that when you drop the weights or set them on the ground, they won't damage your floor.

Dumbbells are great for working out at home. If you don't want to get a gym membership and prefer to work out in privacy, then you may want to consider investing in a dumbbell set. Depending on your fitness level, you don't necessarily need to buy a huge set of these weights. If you are a beginner, you could easily get away with dumbbells up to 30 pounds. If you are further along in your body-conditioning journey, you could start with dumbbells that weigh up to 45 or 50 pounds.

Popular Dumbbell Exercises:

- Bicep curl
- Dumbbell chest press
- Dumbbell fly
- Dumbbell row
- Overhead triceps press
- Triceps kickback
- Walking lunges

Kettle Bells

Kettle bells have become popular in training. Any exercise you can do with dumbbells can be done with kettle bells, but the thicker grip incorporates your forearms more and allows you to be more dynamic with your movements. You can do many types of exercises with kettle bells such as swings and plyometric exercises (moves that are done explosively such as a jump squat or a split squat jump). Kettle bells are often used to do high-repetition sets, such as timed sets for 60 seconds. They help increase the heart rate while simultaneously breaking down muscle tissue. Such exercises are great for breaking through a plateau.

Kettle bells allow you to combine resistance training and cardio training while avoiding having to switch from machine to machine to work your full body. This combination makes for an efficient workout while increasing your core strength. Kettle bells allow you to move through different exercises while challenging your abdominal muscles to keep you stable.

Popular Kettle Bell Exercises:

- Kettle bell dead lift
- Kettle bell push-up
- Kettle bell squat
- Kettle bell swing
- One-arm press with kettle bell
- Power plank row

Barbells

Using barbells allows you to use more resistance because the weight is balanced over the body across a wide length. You will most likely be able to do more repetitions with heavier weights using a barbell than you would with a dumbbell or kettle bell. The more stimulation to your muscles, the better chances of lean muscle tissue growth. The barbell is superior for compound lifts[2] such as the bench press, squat, deadlift, and hang clean that are primarily used to train your major muscle groups.

Barbells also allow you to train for speed, power, coordination, endurance, and can help with fat loss because of the high workload. You will notice when you do barbell exercise programs how much more difficult the workouts feel. This is because it can work three to four muscle groups at a time.

Popular Barbell Lifts:

- Bench press
- Curl
- Deadlift
- Hang clean
- Lunge
- Squat

Cable Machines

Cable machines offer an isolated motion to focus work on specific muscle groups. They are often used to target muscles such as biceps and triceps.

They can be safer than free weights for isolation exercises for someone who is new to working out. The guidance the machines provide on ranges of motion help to reduce the risk of injury.

These machines can also be valuable to someone who needs to balance their bodywork or for someone who is coming back from an injury.

Cable machines are great to supplement your free-weight training and to add to your mix of fitness tools. The movement patterns that can be done with cables are endless, ranging from chest to leg exercises.

Popular Cable Machine Exercises:

- Cable back row
- Cable bicep curl
- Cable chest press
- Cable fly
- Cable hamstring curl
- Cable triceps pushdown

Resistance Training MYTHS

- Resistance training will make a woman look bulky or manly.
- All you need to do is cardio in order to lose weight and maintain weight loss.
- You can spot reduce (reduce the size of just one single area like lower abs or inner thighs).
- High numbers of reps of non-challenging resistance makes you more defined.

Greg's Tips

- Become familiar with the different resistance training tools and try them all.

- Start off light and slow with resistance training, progressively increasing your intensity.

- Track and measure your progress so you can make educated decisions about your resistance-training program.

- Each week increase your weights that you used in the previous week by 2.5 to 5 pounds.

- Change your resistance training routines at least monthly to avoid plateaus. (See chapter on "Putting it Together.")

- Look up three to five new exercises that you have never done before and incorporate them into your workouts for the next week and see how you feel.

- Rest 30 to 60 seconds in between sets, decreasing rest times as your conditioning improves.

- Sleep seven to eight hours per night for maximum recovery.

- See "Exercise Glossary" for descriptions of all exercises described.

CHAPTER SIX

Cardiovascular Fitness

*If you always put limits on everything
you do, physical or anything else, it will
spread into your work and into your
life. There are no limits. There are only
plateaus, and you must not stay there.
You must go beyond them.''*

—Bruce Lee

Why Cardio is Important and How to do It

Cardiovascular training is done by using cardiovascular equipment such as treadmills, stationary bikes, and elliptical machines, or by performing exercises outdoors such as swimming, running, and hiking.

Cardiovascular exercise is important for heart health, for keeping the body lean and toned, and for helping with weight management. There are many misconceptions about how much cardiovascular exercise you should do, how often, and how long you should do it. There are also misconceptions about the benefits of cardiovascular workouts and what they do for the body, especially when it comes to weight loss.

It is very common for cardiovascular exercise to be considered the most important aspect in the fitness journey to lose fat and get toned. In my opinion, though, while vital, it is only *one* part of fitness, not the whole picture. Strength training, nutrition, cardio, core training, stretching, and lifestyle, each play a significant role in your overall fitness. Finding a balance of all of these parts is the key.

In this chapter we will discuss the different types of exercises, the use of cardio equipment, and how to put a cardio program together.

Consult with your physician before starting any exercise program.

Benefits of Cardio Exercise

The benefits of cardio include weight management, fat loss, increased energy levels, reduced stress levels, and heart health. Cardiovascular training makes your heart more efficient. This provides many health benefits such as decreased blood pressure, reduced likelihood of diseases such as heart disease, and reduced stress. Further, cardio exercise improves blood circulation and increases oxygen levels in the blood, which aids the kidneys and liver efficiency in removing toxins that we come into contact with through the environment and the foods we eat.

Cardio exercise can help improve your memory and productivity. The blood that is being pumped into your heart transfers nutrients and oxygen to the brain. Having more oxygen available causes the brain to release hormones that help to increase attention span, perception, and motivation. Studies at the University of Illinois[1] have stated that doing cardio three days per week for sixty minutes increases the size of the hippocampus, the part of the brain that controls memory and learning.

Taking part in activities that boost your heart rate are a great way to increase endorphins, which, in turn, help lower your chances of depression and other mood disorders.

Exercising the heart also helps improve your mood. Taking part in activities that boost your heart rate are a great way to increase endorphins, which, in turn, help lower your chances of depression and other mood disorders. You can think of cardio as a cheap form of therapy!

Heart Rate

Just as with increasing muscle strength, if the goal is to see increased progress, then you must continue to challenge yourself with cardiovascular activities. Heart rate training should be performed progressively. Start at a baseline and then increase the intensity of your workouts every week or two in order to safely train your heart.

In some ways, cardio training is just like school. You wouldn't try to graduate a college-level course when you have been out of school for ten years, without first practicing the fundamentals. View heart rate training the same way. Slow and steady.

The best way to track your heart rate is by using a heart rate monitor. I recommend that my clients purchase both the chest strap and watch. This will allow for more accurate and immediate tracking than using the heart rate monitor on a piece of cardio equipment or by counting your heart beats to the second-hand of a watch.

Keep a workout journal as part of your fitness journal (see "The Missing Link"). Record:

- the type of exercise you did,
- how long you performed your cardiovascular activity,
- your heart rates at various times during the activity (such as after you increased intensity or incline),
- how you felt during the activity, and
- your intensity level.

Be sure to track your heart rates with as much detail as possible to see how you can improve your capacity.

Finding Your Target Heart Rate

There are multiple methods for determining the optimal or "target" heart rate you want to reach during cardiovascular exercise, but many formulas are too generic and are solely based on age. Most don't take into account what your health concerns may be, such as having heart disease or diabetes, or whether you have any injuries or limitations, or whether you are in excellent fitness already. And none of them seem to take into account what you are trying to achieve.

My own research and experience in the fitness industry has led me to use an algorithm for finding individualized target heart rates that is based on heart-rate-training studies done over the last decade.

I have used this algorithm to find my own target heart rate based on my goals, and have used it to adapt my clients' workout programs. It is an amazing way to train for weight loss, endurance, fitness, and vitality.

The huge benefit to using this algorithm is that it helps you determine your own maximum effort. The test is based on *perceived effort*, so whether you are 150 pounds or 400 pounds the test is the same.

The safest way to determine how fast you should be going is by choosing a running, jogging or walking speed that feels like you are pushing yourself enough but that you can sustain for ten minutes without feeling sick. It may take a few days of working out to get a feel for where your sweet spot is, but what you are looking for is heavy breathing and that you are putting in some serious effort but not so much that you feel you can't sustain it for ten minutes.

Conduct the following test:

1. Run/jog/walk at your best intensity for ten minutes, jotting down your heart rate at the end of each minute.

2. Choose your goal from the following options:

- Weight loss– to decrease body weight
- Endurance– to increase cardio capacity (ie: to prepare for a race)
- Fitness– for overall improvement in health

3. Email your heart-rate numbers and goal to me at **greg@fiture. co** (*not* ".com") with the subject line "BodyFit Algorithm."

We will input your information into the algorithm and send your *personalized* plan—with low, target, and maximum heart rates—back to you within 48 hours.

Alternatively, you *can* gauge your maximum heart rate by subtracting your age from 220. For example, if you are thirty-five years old, 220 - 35 = 185 beats per minute. Don't let your heart rate get that high, though. Getting too close to your maximum heart rate is dangerous. This method, of course, doesn't take into account what kind of shape you are currently in (whether you are an advanced athlete or whether you are significantly out of shape), but it does give you an idea of what "average" is for your age.

Thus, using this method, if you are thirty-five years old, 185 is your max heart rate, but you'd want to train with your heart rate around 139 to 157 beats per minute. Keep this in mind as I begin to explain the method of training by heart rate. **When I say, "train at higher heart rates," I mean 75—85 percent of that maximum.**

Working Out by Heart Rate

NOTE: Whenever you read the words "high intensity," remember that it is based on what feels intense *to you* based on *your current fitness level*. Never try to mimic someone else's exact workout program as that can be ineffective at best and dangerous at worst. As always, you can feel intensity in your own body; if you are feeling light-headed, faint, or nauseous, you need to slow down.

In the past, the general recommendation for fat burning has been to jog or cycle while keeping the heart rate in a moderately low range, based on age. Some people still use this method. But, newer studies[2] show that heart rate training is important, and that training at higher heart rates is more effective at weight management and fat loss than training at lower heart-rate levels. This is the training method I use and that I use with my clients and I have found great success with it.

Training at higher heart-rate levels doesn't necessarily mean sprinting. It depends on your conditioning and fitness level. A person who is just starting a workout regime and is out of shape may have a high heart rate just keeping up a consistent walk rhythm, while a conditioned athlete would need to run at a faster rate to keep the heart rate high.

I have used heart-rate training based on the algorithm I describe above over the last three years and have seen people lose large

> *You are only competing against you. There is nothing to worry about because you are in this for the long term. You will develop over time and get better with practice. This does get easier. I promise you that. Remember your "why."*

amounts of weight and become more healthy. In fact, I changed my own cardio work to keep my heart rate at a higher level (a higher intensity) while maintaining the same amount of time I spent on cardio as before. Within one month I lost body fat and significantly increased my fitness level.

My clients have also seen more results by using this training method. I highly recommend that you try it. The overall goal is to burn as many calories from fat as possible while using our time and energy as efficiently as possible. That is why focusing on heart-rate training and duration can be useful for getting more results in less time.

To use this method of cardio training, continually incrementally increase the speed you normally walk, run, or bicycle and increase the intensity by using uphill areas; increase the resistance and speed on a stationary bike or elliptical; and/or increase your incline and speed on the treadmill. Basically, just put more overall effort into the same cardio workout time.

If you are dreading cardio work, remember that the great thing about training in this manner is that *you* have full control of how hard you work and how long you go. Just be sure to track your progress and try to push a little more each time.

You are only competing against you. There is nothing to worry about because you are in this for the long term. You will develop over time and get better with practice. This *does* get easier. I promise you that. Remember your "why."

Frequency of Cardiovascular Exercise

How often you should do cardio is based on your fitness goals. If your fitness goal is to lose weight, then consider increasing your cardio frequency to at least five times per week. If you are focused on improved health purposes or weight maintenance, three to four days a week with a slightly elevated heart rate will help you maintain your current fitness levels. If the goal is to see body composition changes then the more often you perform cardiovascular exercises the better.

By performing cardiovascular exercises during more of your workouts each week you will be able to increase the number of calories your body burns, and keep your metabolism going. By performing cardio exercises more often, you will condition your body for constant effort, which will put it in better shape. This will, in turn, allow you to train more intensely, and create the opportunity for your body to handle more exercise, more intense exercise, and to burn more calories at each exercise.

Keep yourself accountable to doing some kind of cardio every day. Schedule your workout time and stay disciplined. The goal is to make your workout time part of your daily routine, like taking a shower or brushing your teeth.

When doing cardiovascular work, choose from several you

enjoy and frequently change the types of exercises in order to avoid boredom and to keep your body from adapting to the exercise, which reduces results. The constant changing will give your joints and tendons needed rest, which helps avoid overuse and possible injury.

It helps to have a written plan about which exercises you will do each day. The plan will let you better make adjustments and analyze your progress. By closely tracking this work in your fitness journal, you can learn what works best for you and prevent mental burn-out and physical plateaus. It will also allow you to see trends in your behavior, motivation levels, and how well you stick to your schedule. This is valuable information.

Duration of Cardio Exercise

The duration of the cardio section of your workout depends on what your goals are. If you are a competitive runner or want to run distances like 5Ks or marathons then you are going to be running greater distances than if you are focused on being fit and toned.

How long you do your cardio exercises should be based on your intensity of training. Intensity is dictated by how fast you are moving or how high the resistance is to your activity. If you are not using equipment, it will be based on if you are moving uphill or downhill. If you are playing sports, it will be based on how hard you are pushing yourself. The higher the intensity, the shorter the duration.

If your goal is fitness and weight loss, the shortest duration I would recommend is twenty minutes and the maximum is sixty minutes.

Cardio: The Mental Game

People who tend to avoid cardio are those who are new to working out. Let's face it, getting your heart rate up when your heart hasn't been pumping very hard for a long time isn't easy. Pretty much everybody who starts a life-changing program has some anxiety about it.

Think of how good you will look and feel and about all of the benefits you will receive by doing cardio. Think of how it will change your life. Mental talk has a lot to do with this. Thinking about hating cardio won't help and *can* hurt your chances of sustaining your efforts long term. Tell yourself over and over, "I love what cardio is going to do for my body, my health, and my life!" Even if it is hard to get through at first, having a positive mental mantra will help you through it.

> *Think of how good you will look and feel and about all the benefits you will receive by doing cardio.*

Don't think you have to start right off the bat with a super-high-intensity workout to get results. And don't feel like you have to change from where you are to looking like a celebrity in a short amount of time or you are a failure. That is a legitimate belief that a lot of my clients have and I am here to say it is wrong.

Start out easy. Talk with your doctor and consult a trainer to see what a good starting place might be for you. Consider taking an easy walk twice a day, even if it is just for five minutes. If your feet or knees hurt, then start off with a stationary bike or elliptical machine. If those do not work then find a local pool and swim—it is easy on the joints and a great way to begin.

The key is not to build this up too much in your head and put too much pressure on yourself. Start small and progress each week trying to do a little more with a little more intensity.

Keep your eye on your personal progress and not on trying to look like someone else.

Alternative Cardio Options

If you *don't* enjoy cardio then you can adjust how you do your resistance training to give yourself a cardio-like effect. If you take shorter rests in between your sets and incorporate things such as super sets and drop sets (see "Resistance Training"), you can raise your heart rate just as effectively.

> *The key is not to build this up too much in your head and put too much pressure on yourself.*

Besides beginners, the people who tend to dislike cardio are those who are bored easily and think that it can only consist of running on a treadmill or walking for long stretches of time. That is exactly why you will want to plan a variety of activities. Boredom can kill an exercise program. Don't fall into this trap. When thinking about exercise, always visualize the end result and be conscious about why you are working out in the first place.

Consider joining group sports like basketball, football, soccer, or boxing. There are plenty of sports to choose from—broaden your horizons. These kinds of activities focus your mind on an end goal, such as scoring a basket or beating your opponent, which can make the exercise more fun and keep you pushing yourself in ways that solitary exercises like running may not.

Keep your eye on your personal progress and not trying to look like someone else.

Of course, some activities, like basketball, require constant movement while others do not, like baseball. Look for those that do. (No disrespect to baseball—I'm a former player and love the sport!)

If you don't want to be stuck in a gym but aren't able to do group sports, try activities like swimming, rollerblading, or mountain biking.

This isn't an either-or proposition. Try to incorporate many different types of cardio into your lifestyle. There is no single way to accomplish your goals.

Cardio Choices for Injuries

If you have arthritis or are recovering from surgery you have fewer cardio options from which to choose, but you can still actively engage in aerobic exercises. If you have joint problems, exercises such as swimming will be safer and will not irritate your body as much. You can accomplish the same goals as you would running on a treadmill, while reducing the risk of reinjuring yourself or irritating the injured area.

If you have problems or pain in any of your lower body joints, you may find that exercising on a stationary bike or elliptical machine suits you best. These pieces of equipment can give you the same cardio workout as running, without pounding your joints.

Cardio for Bulking Up

During your bulking up phase, don't do cardio activity. If you need to do cardio, keep it minimal: 30 minutes once or twice a week (perhaps short sprints or an incline walk, but nothing overly aerobic). Once you have reached your goal weight, start to incorporate more cardio into your program; transition into the training format I have given for toning up until you reach the body fat percentage that you want.

Cardio for Toning Up

You must increase the heart rate to burn calories. In my experience, the hard part for clients who want to be more toned is realizing that they must put forth a much higher level of intensity in their workouts than they are used to performing.

But again, intensity is relative to what you are currently used to as far as fitness levels are concerned. For example, a client who is 300 pounds and has been living a very sedentary life will find that simply walking around the neighborhood for twenty minutes may be high intensity for that person.

Include cardio in every workout. Cardio activities should be of high intensity for *you* but not require you to overexert. Focus on getting your heart rate up and challenge yourself, but don't overdo.

There are plenty of ways to get the heart rate levels up, but these activities[3] are some of the best:

- Sprint training: running as fast as you can for short bursts followed by short rests

- High-intensity training: using maximum effort separated by longer rest periods (similar to sprint training but longer rest periods)

- Incline walking: walking on an incline of twelve to thirty percent

- Running uphill: running on an incline as part of either sprint training or sustained jogging or walking.

Interval Training

Interval training works both the aerobic and anaerobic energy systems. By training in interval training style, also known as high-intensity training (HIT), your body learns to increase the oxygen to your muscles. The benefits are increased endurance, reduced lactic acid build-up (cramping/fatigue), and being able to train at higher levels of intensity.

Interval training using cardio equipment involves working as hard as you can for one minute on a single cardio machine exercise, followed by one minute doing a passive recovery activity such as walking, then repeating that pattern for 20 minutes.

A benefit of interval training is the opportunity to train a different energy system, which is anaerobic. Interval training can also help burn more calories and build more muscle than only doing cardio, while increasing endurance. Interval training should be used in your overall training scheme to balance out your program two or three times per week. I generally don't recommend more since it is so intense and can cause overtraining.

Interval training also has a mental training component to it. This style of training makes you more mentally tough. When you are performing high-intensity exercises, the body experiences medium to high levels of discomfort, causing you to want to quit. The challenge is to eliminate the negative thoughts in order to achieve the end goal of increased fitness. This teaches you to focus and to push through discomfort. It can also increase your confidence when you get through a HIT workout because you prove to yourself that you can do something that you thought you couldn't.

This confidence can transfer to other areas of your life. It can symbolize the times when life gets hard and you feel like quitting. Completing high-intensity interval training sessions trains your mind to push through the obstacles in life.

Types of Cardio Exercises

These are just examples. Any activity that gets your heart rate up and keeps it up for a period of time will work. My advice is to try many different kinds. Mixing it up will also help you avoid plateaus.

- Bicycling
- Elliptical
- Jogging
- Jumping rope
- Plyometric exercises: exercises done with bursts of energy such as jumping, jump squats, etc.
- Rowing machine
- Shadow boxing
- Sports
- Stair stepper
- Stationary bike
- Treadmill
- Walking
- Zumba class

Treadmill Exercises

Using the treadmill is a great tool for those who enjoy running or walking and don't have any nagging injuries that may become irritated by these activities. The treadmill can be utilized to do incline or decline walking or running. The variations that you can do on the treadmill—besides running and walking forward—are side shuffles, skips, backwards walking, and lunges.

The same principle applies to the treadmill as it does to weights. The more variety, the better and faster your body will respond. The way you control your intensity is by either increasing the speed that you run or walk, or by increasing the incline of the treadmill, or both. There are various programs that are usually pre-installed on the equipment, but I recommend that you just stay on the "Manual" or "Quick Start" setting. You should have full control of your speed and incline and how hard you train based on your heart rate. You want to stay in control of your work out. Keep the moves you use on the treadmill changing so that the workout is dynamic.

Incline Training

In a recent blog post I talked about the benefits of incline training and how it can burn fat and calories in less time. Some newer studies[4] have shown that if you walk at 2.5 to 3 miles per hour on an incline of 18 percent or higher for 20 to 30 minutes, you tap into your fat stores better than by anaerobic running (doing short sprints at maximal effort). This is great news for someone who has ankle or knee problems because fat loss can be achieved without running.

NOTE: Many home-use treadmills only go up to a 15 percent incline. If that's what you have, use it. If or when it is possible, try the incline trainers at your local gym.

Incline Walking Backwards

Walking backwards on a treadmill incorporates more quadriceps recruitment, especially if you stay on your toes. Yes, that's what I said: walk on the balls of your feet, backwards, while the treadmill is set at an incline. Just be careful as you attempt to do this. Set the treadmill at a very slow pace until you get the feel for it. If you can't keep your balance on your toes, just try to keep your weight forward on your feet.

Be sure that you are squatting down, leaning slightly forward to accomplish the most results. Stay in an athletic position. By sitting lower in your walk while going backwards, you strengthen your hamstrings. Walking backwards is also a good way to build up your calf muscles. (See "Exercise Glossary" for a visual of this activity.)

We don't usually walk backwards in day-to-day living, so by doing it you get a chance to work a different part of your body and balance your muscles. Muscle imbalances can cause injuries to the back and hamstrings. (See more about muscle imbalance in "Resistance Training.")

Skipping

Skipping on the treadmill can build strength in your core while activating the nervous system because it is a coordination exercise. The more you get the nervous system involved in your exercise, the more you can tap into your fat stores. Also, skipping on the treadmill is a great way to challenge your body in new ways.

Side Shuffles

Side shuffles on the treadmill are great for not only increasing your heart rate and strengthening leg muscles but also for building the oblique region of the core abdominals. Since it is not a common movement to shuffle side-to-side, it can challenge the cardiovascular system more than running or walking forward. Side-to-side shuffles also help keep the body more balanced. Because of the sideways push, the gluteus (hips and buttocks) muscles are used and strengthened, making this is a great way to build more firm and shapely gluteus and hamstrings.

How to Perform Side Shuffles

Standing sideways on the treadmill, with your right leg toward the front end of the treadmill, take your first step with your right foot, then bring your left foot next to your right foot (almost touching) and then repeat. You should stay on the balls of your feet, keeping your core tight and controlling your body.

Lunges

Doing lunges on a treadmill is a new experience. You have to slow the treadmill down to 1.5 miles per hour so that you can control the movement. The lunge on an incline (15 percent incline or higher—the higher the better) is the most effective exercise to do if you are trying to get deeper hamstring and gluteus recruitment. The incline lunge is a great exercise to incorporate as a super set (performing two exercises with no rest) with weight training for legs. It also raises the heart rate effectively.

How to Perform a Lunge

When doing lunges, keep your body in an upright position with your core tight. As you lunge forward, make sure your knee lines up over your toes. Never go past your toes, in order to avoid injury.

Elliptical

Elliptical training is great for those who have knee problems and cannot take the pounding of running on the treadmill. The elliptical is a piece of cardio equipment that mimics the running motion but takes the stress off the body because it uses a gliding motion, with the feet never leaving the pedals. There are different types of elliptical machines. Some have handles for the arms, while other don't. Choose one that is the most comfortable for you. They both accomplish the same result. (The machines that have arm handles don't really help you burn more calories to make a huge difference.)

Controlling the intensity of the elliptical is based on resistance. In order to keep seeing results, increase the resistance progressively every week. Also, use backward motion as well as the forward motion for total leg development.

Stationary Bike

The stationary bike helps develop the leg muscles and increase endurance. Leg and muscle endurance happen when your muscles can sustain repeated resistance over a longer time.

The stationary bike puts minimal stress on the joints. If you are at the beginning of your fitness journey, this is a great piece of equipment for you. The best way to increase your results on the bike is to increase the resistance, just like with the elliptical trainer. Set the seat where it feels comfortable—about the height of your hip—and make sure that your knees are not going past the line of your toes. You should be able to pedal comfortably without having to fully extend your leg or create any extra movements to help. There should be a natural and smooth flow.

Start slowly and increase both resistance and speed progressively by one level or point each week to consistently challenge your body.

This is a great exercise to set based on heart rate, so get a heart rate monitor to track your intensity.

Stationary bikes come with and without backrests. The differences are based on riding intensity. If you are a more intense rider and are trying to elevate your heart rate as high as possible, you will want to ride the bike without the back support. The bikes with back support are good for people who have back problems and for people rehabilitating injuries.

Swimming

Swimming is a workout that you can use to help build up tendons and joints while improving your cardio fitness. Swimming can be challenging if you do not have good form, but once you learn how to be efficient in your stroke, swimming can elevate your heart rate. The benefits of swimming include a total body workout—particularly core, shoulder, and back strengthening.

Swimming workouts such as sprints or full-effort body movements are beneficial because the water adds resistance to the movements. If you have joint problems or injury tendency, pool work is a good choice because you experience resistance with minimal stress on the joints.

Running

Running outside is a pastime of many exercisers, and is a fantastic way to get in shape. Getting the heart rate up is the name of the game, and if you purchase a heart monitor and track your heart rate you can maximize your runs.

Running shoes are also important since you are running on hard ground and there is no padding to absorb the shock. Buy a quality pair of running shoes with a good sole that can take some wear and tear. The shoes should also form to your feet comfortably. Consider consulting with a shoe company or store that specializes in helping runners get the best shoes and soles for competition. This is a worthwhile investment that should allow you to run longer with fewer injuries.

Kickboxing

Kickboxing builds muscle definition in the abdominals and core but also increases your cardio as well. Kickboxing is a good cardio exercise because it requires the full body at full intensity to perform. Your body will burn more calories and requires more energy to do the movements than doing exercises that only work one muscle group at a time, such as a single leg extension. A good kickboxingclasscannotonlygiveyouagoodworkoutbutteachyouself-defense skills, too.

Jump Rope

Jumping rope is a favorite of boxers and fighters because it involves a full-body workout and requires good coordination. The way you control jump rope intensity is by doing speed rope. The goal is to do as many reps (jumps) as possible in an allotted time.

A good challenge is twelve sets of jumping for three minutes, with one minute of rest in between each set.

The intensity of jumping rope will give you results in strength, endurance, and productive body-fat burn. Some variations that you can add to your jump-rope routine are one-leg jumps, double skipping, side-to-side, and alternating feet.

Rowing

The rowing machine is a way to strengthen back muscles. By keeping the resistance low, you may sustain the exercise for long periods of time, which can increase your endurance. The lower the resistance, the faster you can go, and the more likely you will reach an aerobic state. According to the United States of Rowing, this activity can burn up to 500 calories in an hour.

Greg's Tips

- Check with your physician before starting any exercise program.

- Choose cardio activities that you enjoy and do a mix of different activities each week.

- Purchase a heart rate monitor for optimum results.

- Create a workout journal as part of your fitness journal, to track your progress and heart rates.

- Interchange your cardio workouts between aerobic and anaerobic.

CHAPTER SEVEN

Putting It Together

*Anything worthwhile
didn't happen overnight.*

– G.M.

This chapter is about how you build your lifestyle of fitness using all of the tools we've talked about in previous chapters. Let's piece it together sequentially.

Cycles of Betterment

The FITT Principle

We've talked about the importance of increasing the intensity of your workouts a little each day, and incrementally each week, in both cardio and resistance training. And we've talked about changing your workout pattern or program at least once a month.

The system that you can use to make these changes is the **FITT Principle**. It stands for frequency, intensity, time, and type. These are the four ways you can switch up your workout programs to continuously stay out of the plateau region and keep yourself challenged.

Frequency:

Increase how many times per week or month you work out.

Intensity:

Increase how hard you exercise by the speed of your cardio or how level of resistance during strength training.

Time:

Increase how long you do a single cardio exercise. In resistance training, increase the number of sets per exercise you do and/or move to more difficult types of lifts.

Type:

Change the activities and exercises in your workouts.

These are the key components to consider when you want to progress your training program to the next level. By understanding these fundamentals, you have a systematic way to meet your fitness goals.

The Long Haul

Now I want to talk about the long haul. This is a lifestyle change. Don't look at it as, "I have to work out until I obtain this goal, then I can stop," because, for one thing, you won't maintain the results of your goal and all of that hard work.

So how do you keep from getting bored with a lifetime of staying fit and healthy? Continue to progress and change your focus. Boredom kills workout plans, so we want to keep your workouts feeling new and interesting.

If you are working toward a specific goal, it may take you more than three months to get there. But when you've hit your stride, a change of focus every three months is the perfect way to mix things up mentally and physically to keep your exercise program feeling fresh, invigorating, and exciting. Doing so also helps you to avoid the dreaded plateau.

Think of it as four cycles of focus each year. One cycle can be for strength, the next can be for toning, or muscular endurance, or aerobic endurance. There is always a way to progress. When you are changing your focus to aerobic endurance, for example, you would do more cardio and a bit less resistance work. It gives your brain a chance to focus on a new goal and keeps your muscles challenged by going a slightly different direction with your workouts.

Eating and Workouts

You have been given *a lot* of information on working out and nutrition to digest (so to speak). If you are reading this through for the first time, it may all seem a little daunting. So I've put some starting courses together for you that bring things together. I'll walk you through the process of what to eat and when to eat in relation to your workouts, as well as take you step by step through how those workouts should be run and what they can incorporate.

I'm also going to simplify how to put your own workouts together once you've got a rhythm going.

Pre-Workout Eating

Your schedule will dictate when you exercise, but there is a prime time and recommended types of foods to eat before and after your workout that will help you attain your goals. Consider when your workouts fit into your day when you are planning your meals. (Note: a pre- or post-workout snack or meal counts toward your total snacks and meals for the day, it isn't in addition to them.)

If you have a pre-workout *snack* I suggest it be eaten about an hour before. If you wake up early in order to work out before your day begins, you can eat immediately before you work out, as long as your stomach can handle it.

Good pre-workout snacks:

- High-protein (20 or more grams protein) granola bar with two cups of grapes
- Yogurt with real fruit mixed into it
- Hummus and crackers
- Half of a peanut butter and honey sandwich on whole wheat bread

For pre-workout *meals* I recommend eating roughly one or two hours before your workout. You want to have fuel, but you don't want to feel full when you are working out. A good pre-workout meal would be something that you can digest easily: mostly healthy carbohydrates mixed with about 20 grams of protein

On the other hand, you don't want to have gone too long without eating. The big mistake I see people make before they exercise is that their last meal was four or even five hours before their workout. When these clients exercise they can't train as hard as they should because their blood sugar drops so low that they feel light-headed. One of the important aspects of getting results is training intensely, and to train intensely your body must have fuel. Pay attention to your pre-workout meals and/or snacks.

Refer to the information in my nutrition chapters. They will help you plan and put meals together that will meet your dietary needs based on your goals.

Your Work Outs–Step by Step[1]

Note: Working Out With An Injury

If you have an injury, modify your workouts. Don't avoid exercising. You want to be respectful of the injury that you have, but not let it slow down your momentum when you are trying to get results. Sometimes injuries happen and you just have to work around them methodically.

For example, when I broke my leg, it was close to eight months before I could start running and performing as usual again. Even though my leg was broken and I was in a cast, I didn't let that stop me from lifting weights and even doing cardio exercises. I trained my upper body each day and pushed it to the maximum, and I rode the stationary bike with my cast. It didn't cause me pain and I didn't put too much pressure on my body. I also checked with my doctor about my intended workout program.

Some steps to take if you have an injury or if you are still in the healing process are:

- See your doctor to make sure that you are cleared to exercise. Safety is first and you want to avoid any chance of prolonging your injury or making your injury worse.

- Establish what your goals are and what your possible limitations are.

- Find exercises that work within your limitations that still provide resistance and cardio as effectively as possible.

- Keep making adjustments as needed and continue to track your progress.

By working around your injury, you will feel much better about your fitness journey because you will have maintained a sense of progress. This will also help you deal with your injury better mentally.

Note: Breathing

The importance of breathing during your workouts cannot be emphasized enough. While exercising, maintain a natural breathing pattern. When doing resistance exercises, breathe out at the point of contraction and breathe in at the point of relaxation/elongation.

Just remember you should *never* hold your breath while exercising—it makes it hard to breathe!

Step 1: Warm-up

Do not ever skip the warm-up.

Warming up is essential to preparing your body for exercise. Do thirty-second sets each of full body movements such as lunges, body weight squats, push-ups, ab twists, and supermans. Perform the warm-up exercises in a controlled fashion and be sure to feel it in your muscles.

Start slowly and increase speed and intensity as your body warms and heart rate increases. Never start these warm-up activities at full speed.

Your warm-up should last for about ten minutes. You can perform the exercises in rounds. For example, if you are doing lunges, squats, jump squats, jumping jacks, and push-ups as your rounds, then do each exercise for thirty seconds, repeating them in order for ten minutes. Or alternatively, you could do one minute of each exercise, followed by five minutes of cardio. Either way, the goal is to warm up the whole body.

Step 2: Resistance Exercises

To start, choose three to five resistance exercises that you can do comfortably for a set of twelve to fifteen reps. Perform one to three sets of each exercise, resting thirty to ninety seconds between sets, based on your current fitness levels.

Step 3: Abs

Choose three or four exercises. Do three one-minute sets of each. You should give your abs a day of rest in between workouts. For example, if you work your abs on Monday, don't do focused exercises on the abs again until Wednesday.

Step 4: Cardiovascular exercises

The purpose of your cardio work is to keep your heart rate up so you get a chance to take advantage of your body's natural fat burning zone. Choose cardio exercises that you enjoy and keep you injury-free.

Start off slowly by performing the exercise you have chosen at a very comfortable pace, whether it is running, jumping rope, or walking. Start out doing your cardio exercise for ten to fifteen minutes. This will assess where you are physically, and avoid overtraining in the beginning. The best way to gauge when you are ready for an increase in your workout is how quickly your body recovers from soreness (fast = one day or less; long = two to three days) and how fast your heart rate recovers (fast = five to ten minutes; long = fifteen minutes or more).

The goal is to work up to performing twenty minutes of intense cardio work (based on your goals[2]) and continually ratcheting up the intensity (walking to walking incline to jogging to running at increasing speeds and inclines).

One of the most common mistakes beginners make—and even experienced athletes who haven't been working out for a while—is not controlling their ambition and start off doing too much too fast. The result is becoming too sore to stick with your exercise program.

No matter what kind of resistance training exercises you did, almost any kind of cardio will work, as most cardio relies on the legs to increase the heart rate. You can use whatever cardio activity works for you, but try to mix it up.

Step 5: Active Recovery

There are two types of recovery when it comes to exercising. The first type is active recovery. The second type, passive recovery, I'll discuss later.

Active recovery is effective for getting rid of muscle soreness by the use of lower intensity exercises. These exercises include light cardio activities such as low-intensity stationary bike, walking, doing very low-resistance training, or by keeping any exercise effort to a minimum.

The benefits of active recovery are crucial for the overall development of your fitness program and your body. Active recovery allows you to bounce back faster from your workouts, particularly if they were more intense than your normal exercise routine.

Active recovery is part of your cool-down period between your cardio work and stretching time. After intense cardio, this is a time to slowly lower your heart rate. If you were jogging, don't just stop and hold still. Continually slow the jogging into a walk. Usually the heart rate will sufficiently recover within five minutes or so.

Note: beginners who are building up their workout program can also use active recovery techniques. Alternate days of "intense workouts" with days of "active-recovery workouts." The latter would be days when you do very light exercise, allowing your body to heal, but still getting the muscles warm and moving. Doing this really helps get rid of soreness as you are getting your body used to increased activity.

Step 6: Stretching and Mental Affirmation

Drink plenty of water and stretch.

The importance of stretching is oftentimes overlooked because the perceived benefits of it don't directly translate into better muscular definition, but it is an important step for staying limber and in aiding recovery.

Stretching after your workout is a great way to cool down the muscles and enhance the benefits of your workout by also helping to relieve stress. Practice controlled deep breathing (inhaling through the nose, exhaling through the mouth) and do some mental training and meditation with it.

Visualize the results that you want to obtain and give yourself positive affirmation for the effort you just put forth. Give yourself credit for finishing a workout and doing what it takes to get control of your health. Think about all of the benefits you are getting—and will continue to get—by exercising regularly. Think about the positive emotions you will experience when you reach your goals.

Stretch your muscles gently and slowly. Don't rush. Take your time moving into the full stretch and stop as soon as you feel a slight tightness. Hold the stretch for thirty to sixty seconds. Stretching should feel comfortable; you should not experience any discomfort or pain. If you do, you can cause an injury—stop immediately and apply less pressure to your stretch.

Your stretching time should last around ten to fifteen minutes, but take as long as you need.

You may choose which stretching exercises to do, but try to do at least one for every muscle group. This is the order I prefer:

- Hamstring stretch
- Quadriceps stretch
- Groin stretch
- Hip flexor stretch
- Calf stretch
- IT-band stretch
- Abdominal stretch
- Lower back stretch
- Chest stretch
- Back stretch
- Neck stretch
- Shoulder stretch
- Upper back stretch

Step 7: Post-Workout Eating

Immediately post-workout, have a **snack** to quickly replenish your muscles and start the repair process. Right after your workout your body needs quality nutrition to increase lean muscle tissue.

Good post workout snacks:

- A glass of chocolate milk
- Protein shake with a piece of fruit
- Half of a grilled- or baked-chicken sandwich

Then, **eat a full meal within the hour or two after your work-out** to put some nutrients in your body to expedite your recovery. Recovery is extremely important because the faster you recover (or feel no more soreness) the faster you can work out intensely again.

Your post-workout meal may be one of the most important meals of the day, so a balanced meal with protein and carbohydrates is crucial. You will want to eat roughly 50 grams of carbohydrates and 15 to 20 grams of protein.

Good post workout meals:

- Fish and vegetables
- Steak and vegetables
- Lean hamburger on a wheat bun

Protein is vital to have right after your workouts because it helps to replace glycogen stores, which will help to build more lean muscle tissue.

Any of the meals and snacks in my sample nutrition plan (earlier in this chapter) would be appropriate for pre- or post-workout.

One of the major complaints of exercise programs is how sore people get either the next day or two days later when they perform the prescribed workout program. The two best ways to help alleviate that problem are: 1) to perform active recovery, and 2) I recommend using the supplement glutamine or making sure you are eating foods high in this amino acid.

Foods that have glutamine are meats and seafood, beans, spinach, parsley, and dairy. If you want to boost your intake and choose a supplement, check with your physician and follow the instructions on the label to see how much and when you should take it.

Step 8: Passive Recovery

The second form of recovery, which is called **passive recovery**, is more traditional—almost everyone has at some point just wanted to sit around and rest after a hard work out!

Sleeping is the most common form of passive recovery and while I don't recommend sleeping *immediately* after a work out, getting a good night's sleep is crucial to the functioning of your body.

Workout Routines

Now that you have a handle on just how the whole process works, let me give you some sample routines. My Six-Day Jump-Start Workout Program is, obviously, a great place to start.

It will work for you whether you are a beginner or already in shape. If you are a beginner, start easy with these exercises, watching your form carefully and using light weights for the first week or so, then incrementally increase your speed and resistance. If you are in shape, make sure you are pushing your intensity level with each day.

As I said before, you can use this plan for about a month, then switch up the exercises and layouts of your program using the Build-Your-Own-Workout Menu and by using the FITT principle.

Six-Day Jump-Start Workout Program

Day 1: Chest and Triceps

Warm up:

1 minute each:

- Jumping jacks
- Walking lunge
- Push-ups (can be on knees)
- Body weight squat
- Jump squat

Jog, 5 minutes

Resistance Training:

Bench press or chest press machine: 1—2 sets of 12 reps

Incline bench press: 1—2 sets of 12 reps

Push-ups: 1—2 drop sets

Rope triceps push-down: 1—2 sets of 12 reps

Bench dips: 1—2 sets of 12 reps

Regular ab crunches: 1—2 drop sets

Cardio:

30 minutes: any cardio activity

Stretch:

While you are stretching, breath in slowly through the nose, exhale through the mouth and mentally repeat your "Why" and imagine me giving you a high five! "Great work today! You did it!"

About 10–15 minutes (in this order):

Hamstring stretch

Quadriceps stretch

Groin stretch

Hip flexor stretch

Calf stretch

IT-band stretch

Abdominal stretch

Lower back stretch

Chest stretch

Back stretch

Neck stretch

Shoulder stretch

Upper back stretch

Day 2: Back and Biceps

Warm up:

Stationary bike, 5 minutes

1 minute each:

- Side shuffles
- Step-ups
- Burpees
- Arm circles
- Plank

Resistance Training:

Lat pull-down: 1—2 sets of 12 reps

Seated row: 1—2 sets of 12 reps

Deadlift: 1—2 sets of 12 reps

EZ curl bicep curl: 1—2 sets of 12 reps

Preacher bicep curl: 1—2 sets of 12 reps

Regular ab crunches: 1—2 drop sets

Cardio:

30 minutes: any cardio activity

Stretch:

While you are stretching, breath in slowly through the nose, exhale through the mouth and mentally repeat your "Why" and imagine me congratulating you, "Wow! Way to push yourself!"

About 10—15 minutes (in this order):

Hamstring stretch

Quadriceps stretch

Groin stretch

Hip flexor stretch

Calf stretch

IT-band stretch

Abdominal stretch

Lower back stretch

Chest stretch

Back stretch

Neck stretch

Shoulder stretch

Upper back stretch

Day 3: Legs

Warm up:

Elliptical, 5 minutes

1 minute each:

- Ab twist
- Skip

- Side step-ups
- Stationary lunge
- Split squat jumps

Resistance Training:

Squats: 1—2 sets of 12 reps

Stationary lunge: 1—2 sets of 12 reps

Step-ups: 1—2 sets of 12 reps

Seated calf-raise: 1—2 sets of 12 reps

Regular ab crunches: 1—2 drop sets

Cardio:

30 minutes: any activity

Stretch:

While you are stretching, breath in slowly through the nose, exhale through the mouth and mentally repeat your "Why" and "Now *that's* what I'm talkin' about!"

About 10—15 minutes (in this order):

Hamstring stretch

Quadriceps stretch

Groin stretch

Hip flexor stretch

Calf stretch

IT-band stretch

Abdominal stretch

Lower back stretch

Chest stretch

Back stretch

Neck stretch

Shoulder stretch

Upper back stretch

Day 4: Shoulders

Warm up:

Walk, incline treadmill 5—10%, 6 minutes

Incline treadmill 5—10%, 1 minute each:

- Side shuffle right
- Side shuffle left
- Lunge
- Backwards walk on balls of feet

Resistance Training:

Shoulder press: 1—2 sets of 12 reps

Lateral raise: 1—2 sets of 12 reps

Front raise: 1—2 sets of 12 reps

Upright row: 1—2 sets of 12 reps

Regular abdominal crunches: 1—2 drop sets

Cardio:

30 minutes: any activity

Stretch:

While you are stretching, breath in slowly through the nose, exhale through the mouth and mentally repeat your "Why" and "Woo-hoo! That was some SERIOUSLY impressive effort!"

About 10—15 minutes (in this order):

Hamstring stretch

Quadriceps stretch

Groin stretch

Hip flexor stretch

Calf stretch

IT-band stretch

Abdominal stretch

Lower back stretch

Chest stretch

Back stretch

Neck stretch

Shoulder stretch

Upper back stretch

Day 5: Cardio & Abs

Warm up:

10 minutes, Stationary bike

Resistance Training:

Regular ab crunches: 1—2 drop sets

Bicycles: 1—2 sets of 12 reps

Reverse crunch: 1—2 sets of 12 reps

Cardio:

30-45 minutes, a single cardio activity of choice

Stretch:

While you are stretching, breath in slowly through the nose, exhale through the mouth and mentally repeat your "Why" and "SAH-WEET workout! You came today with your game face on!"

About 10—15 minutes (in this order):

Hamstring stretch

Quadriceps stretch

Groin stretch

Hip flexor stretch

Calf stretch

IT-band stretch

Abdominal stretch

Lower back stretch

Chest stretch

Back stretch

Neck stretch

Shoulder stretch

Upper back stretch

Day 6: Cardio

Warm up:

10 minutes, Stationary bike

Cardio:

30 minute: any activity

Stretch:

While you are stretching, breath in slowly through the nose, exhale through the mouth and mentally repeat your "Why" and "Look how tough you are! You pushed through an AMAZING week! Congratulations!"

About 10—15 minutes (in this order):

Hamstring stretch

Quadriceps stretch

Groin stretch

Hip flexor stretch

Calf stretch

IT-band stretch

Abdominal stretch

Lower back stretch

Chest stretch

Back stretch

Neck stretch

Shoulder stretch

Upper back stretch

Build Your Own Workout

If you've used the Six-Day Jump Start Program for a while, you are getting used to the various activities and exercises. This system should help you take the next step in your training and let you create whatever you think you need to get to the next level of fitness.

I'd like to see you working out at least five days a week. Every other day would have resistance and cardio training, the remaining two would include mainly stretching. As soon as you feel up for it, add cardio to your stretching days as well. I like you to start off with frequent cardio sessions to get your body accustomed to exercising every day. The goal is to make a habit of working out five to six days per week. Increasing slowly will get your body prepared to progress to more intermediate and advanced workouts while minimizing your risk for injury.

Here is how a day would look (use this with the Build-Your-Own-Workout Menu).

Monday:

Warm up, 5—10 minutes

Resistance, 20—30 min. (focus: chest, triceps; 2—4 exercises
per muscle group)

Cardio, 20—30 minutes

Stretch, 10—15 minutes

Tuesday:

Warm up, 5—10 minutes

Cardio, 20—30 minutes

Stretch, 20—30 minutes

Wednesday:

Warm up, 5—10 minutes

Resistance, 20—30 minutes (focus: back, biceps; 2—4 exercises per muscle group)

Cardio, 20—30 minutes

Stretch, 10—15 minutes

Thursday:

Warm up, 5—10 minutes

Cardio, 20–30 minutes

Stretch, 20–30 minutes

Friday:

Warm Up, 5–10 minutes

Resistance, 20–30 minutes (focus: legs, shoulders; 2-4 exercises per muscle group)

Cardio, 20–30 minutes

Stretch, 10–15 minutes

If/when you are able to add another day:

Saturday:

Warm up, 5–10 minutes

Cardio, 20–30 minutes

Stretch, 20–30 minutes

Although it isn't ideal, there are times when we can't fit five days of workouts into a week, and some people have schedules that make this extremely difficult. For those times, consider these programs:

Four-Day Program

Day 1: Warm up, Legs and Abs, Cardio, Stretch

Day 2: Warm up, Chest and Triceps, Cardio, Stretch

Day 3: Warm up, Back and Abs & Biceps, Cardio, Stretch

Day 4: Warm up, Shoulders, Cardio, Stretch

Three-Day Program

Day 1: Warm up, Legs, Abs, Cardio, Stretch

Day 2: Warm up, Chest and Back, Cardio, Stretch

Day 3: Warm up, Arms and Shoulders & Abs, Cardio, Stretch

The adjustments needed to make a change for each person's schedule generally comes down to making sure that you workout each muscle group at least once a week and aim to do cardio on each workout day as well.

If you can't do cardio every day because it is too difficult, then do cardio every other day. The same applies with weight training. Make sure that the body is getting built up to the activity and use your body as a gauge to tell you if you are pushing yourself too hard too fast.

Build-Your-Own-Workout Menu

Building a workout isn't entirely unlike choosing items from a take-out menu—except *this* is a healthy menu. You want to choose a bit from each of the columns to get a nice balance of flavors, or, in this case, physical activity. So instead of a take-out menu, here is your workout menu.

Follow this routine for four weeks, then switch things up. But remember to increase intensity each day by at least a little bit, to avoid that plateau.

As you are learning the exercises in the beginning, be sure to refer to the "Exercise Glossary" to make sure your stance is correct and that your contraction positions are neither too short nor over-extended.

Build-Your-Own Workout Menu

Total Workout Time: about one hour

WARM UP

- Choose 5 exercises
- Do each for 1 minute
- Add 5 minutes cardio

OR

- Choose 5 exercises
- Do each for 30 seconds, repeat

EXERCISES:

Ab twists

Body-weight squats

Burpee

Jogging

Jumping jacks

Kettle bell swing

Lunges

Power push press

Push-ups

Supermans

Thigh blasters

Walking

RESISTANCE

- Choose 3—5 exercises.
- Do 1—3 sets of 12—15 reps.
- Rest 30—90 seconds between sets.

(See Resistance Exercises Menu)

As you become more comfortable with putting workouts together, refer back to the other chapters for other exercise options and combinations for both cardio and resistance training.

ABDOMINALS:

- Every OTHER Day
- Choose 3—4 exercises.
- Do 3 one-minute sets of each exercise

Ab crunch
- Bicycle
- Bosu ball
- Decline
- Exercise ball
- Medicine ball
- Oblique
- Physioball
- Regular
- Reverse
- Roman chair lift

Ab twist

Hanging leg raise

Kettle bell power plank row

Plank

Push-up (regular)

Sit-up

CARDIO

- About 20 minutes, depending on your goals
- Follow with active recovery exercises until heart rate recovers.

Home:

Walking

Jogging

Plyometric exercises

Jumping rope

Shadow boxing

Bicycling

Active sports like soccer or basketball that keep you moving.

Gym:

Treadmill

Elliptical

Stationary bike

Zumba class

Rowing machine

Stair stepper

STRETCH

- Stretch 10—15 min. or until your full body is stretched
- Go slowly; never stretch far enough to cause discomfort
- Breathe deeply and slowly
- Think about your 'Why'
- Choose a mantra that helps support your goals and repeat it!

Hamstring stretch

Quadriceps stretch

Groin stretch

Hip Flexor stretch

Calf stretch

IT-band stretch

Abdominal stretch

Lower back stretch

Chest stretch

Back stretch

Neck stretch

Shoulder stretch

Upper back stretch

Resistance Exercises Menu

- Choose 3—5 exercises.

- Do 1—3 sets of 12—15 reps each

- Rest 30—90 seconds between sets, depending on your workout goals

NOTE:
See "Exercise Glossary" for definition of terms

ARMS

Arm circle

Cable curl

Dumbbell overhead press

Kettle bell one-arm press

Kettle bell push-up

Pull-up

Push-up

Row, seated or upright

(Bicep):

Curl
- Barbell
- Dumbbell
- Forearm/wrist

Hammer

Preacher

Resistance band
- Back row
- Bicep curl

(Triceps):

Bed dip

Cable pushdown

Chair dip

Dumbbell chest press
- Dumbbell kickback

Pushdown
- Cable
- Regular
- Rope

Resistance band extension

Shoulder press

Skull crusher

Triceps kickback

SHOULDERS

Bed dip

Chair dip

Hang clean

Hammer-strength chest press

Front raise

Kettle bell one-arm press

Kettle bell push-up

Lateral raise

Pull-up

Push-up

Rear deltoid raise

Resistance band shoulder raise

Shoulder press

CHEST

Bench press

Cable chest press

Cable fly

Chair dip

Chest Press
  • Dumbbell
  • Machine

Dumbbell fly

Hammer strength

Kettle bell push-up

Push-up

FULL BODY

Burpee

Jumping jacks

Kettle bell swing

Power push press

BACK

Deadlift (lower back)

Hang clean

Lat pull-down

Pull-up

Row
  • Cable
  • Dumbbell
  • Seated
  • Kettle bell power plank
  • Upright

Superman (lower back)

LEGS

Cable hamstring curl

Calf machines

Calf raise

Leg
  • Curl (hamstring)
  • Extension (quad)

Press (quad, hamstring)

Lunge (quad, hamstring)
  • Dumbbell
  • Dumbbell walking
  • Regular
  • Walking
  • Stationary
  • Treadmill

Resistance band side shuffle

Side shuffles

Squat (quad, hamstring)
  • Body weight
  • Dumbbell
  • Jump
  • Kettle bell
  • Split squat jump

Standing calf raise

Step-up (regular, side)

Thigh blaster (quad)

Treadmill

Lunges

Side shuffles

Walking backward incline

Bulking Up vs. Toning Up Review

I have offered details throughout the chapters on how to use resistance training, cardio, nutrition, and supplements to bulk up or to tone up your body. Here is an overview, putting all of the information together.

Bulking Up Review

Nutrition for Bulking Up

- Increase caloric intake by 500 calories per day be eating good, whole, healthy foods.

- Eat 1 to 1 1/2 grams of protein per pound of body weight per day.

- Keep a daily food journal.

- Drink plenty of water.

Resistance Training for Bulking Up

- Focus your workouts on compound exercises such as the bench press and squat.

- Lift the heaviest weights you can for sets of five to eight reps. This assumes that you already have a workout in place. If you don't, start the first few weeks with lighter weights and slowly work your way up to the heavy ones.

- Lift the weights in a controlled fashion without arching your back or locking out your knees or elbows.

- Make sure that you focus your effort on using the desired muscle group.

- Only work out one or two major muscle groups per day, then give those muscle groups a rest and focus on others the next day.

Cardio for Bulking Up

- None. Or no more than 30 minutes of light cardio once or twice a week.

- Once you have reached your goal weight, start to incorporate more cardio into your program.

Rest for Bulking Up

One of the most important tools for gaining muscle mass is rest. You want to keep your body in an anabolic state, so the more sleep you get, the better your body will recover and the more results you will see.

I recommend seven to nine hours of sleep per night. Also get yourself in a routine of falling asleep at the same time each night so it becomes easier for you to get quality sleep.

Sleep isn't the only form of rest that I recommend. Also make sure you are getting one or two days of rest from any working out (resistance or cardio) each week. Eventually you can work out at this level five days a week, but I wouldn't do more than that at this level.

Because your level of intensity is so high you must be careful not to over-train. Doing so will put you in a muscle wasting state, which will seriously reduce your ability to get the results you want. So I cannot overemphasize the importance of rest.

Supplements for Bulking Up

Always consult a physician before using any supplements, as the FDA does not monitor them, and follow the instructions on the bottle. Some supplements to consider for bulking up:

- Multi-vitamin
- Creatine (take about two hours before you lift weights)
- Glutamine before and after your workouts (as per label)
- Whey protein (about an hour before and immediately after your workout)
- Combine casein protein with your meals—especially with whole food proteins
- NOTE: If you are lactose intolerant try rice, soy, or beef protein powders instead of whey or casein proteins.
- Fish oils throughout the day

Toning Up Review

Nutrition for Toning Up

- Reduce caloric intake by 500 calories per day, if weight loss is necessary.

- Especially because you are reducing calories, take care that the calories you do consume come from good, whole, healthy foods.

- Eat 1 gram of protein per pound of body weight each day from lean sources like fish, chicken, and turkey.

- Keep a daily detailed food journal.

- Drink plenty of water.

- Eat four to five times per day (three meals and one or two snacks).

- Eat most of your carbohydrates in the morning.

- Eat high quality fats such as olive oil, fish oil, nuts, and/ or flaxseed oil, while minimizing carbohydrate intake to fist-sized portions per meal (or smaller, depending on your energy and whether you are achieving your desired results).

Resistance Training for Toning Up

- Exercise five or six days per week for best results.

- Generally, choose one or two muscle groups to focus on per workout (for variety and muscle confusion you can incorporate full-body workouts into your routine).

- Focus on doing exercises that work large muscle groups such as squats, bench presses, back rows, and shoulder presses.

- Perform 30- to 60-minute workouts including three or four resistance exercises. Perform two or three sets of 10 to 15 reps for each exercise and rest very minimally (if at all) between sets.

Cardio for Toning Up

- Include cardio in every workout (15 minutes minimum; 60 minutes maximum).

- Cardio activities should be of high intensity (remember this intensity is what feels like an effort for *you*: get the heart rate up to a level that is challenging but not over-exerting).

Rest for Toning Up

Rest is crucial for getting the results that you want. The more rest you get, the better your body will recover, and the more energy you will have to do more intense workouts.

Because you are exercising intensely, getting enough rest should not be overlooked (as it often is). I suggest sleeping seven to nine hours per night and creating a sleep routine (same time each night) so it is easier to fall asleep and get quality sleep. Be sure to have at least one full rest day where you don't do anything, so your body can recover and you can go into the next week of your workouts with full intensity.

Supplements for Toning Up

Always consult a physician before using any supplements, as the FDA does not monitor them, and follow the instructions on the bottle. Some supplements to consider for toning up:

- Multi-vitamin
- Whey protein (about an hour before and immediately after your workout).

- Combine casein protein with your meals—especially with whole food proteins.
- NOTE: If you are lactose intolerant try rice, soy, or beef protein powders instead of whey or casein proteins.
- Fish oils throughout the day

Greg's Thoughts

- Be patient with your results and constantly tweak your strategy for getting the results you want. Really pay attention to your form and how your body feels.
- Keep up the great work you are doing. The best thing you can do for your life is to be proactive with your health. You are part of an elite group of people who are taking control of their destiny. I'm proud of you.

Exercise Glossary & Workout Terminology

List of Exercises by Major Muscle Groups

Arms (biceps, triceps)

Arm circle
Bicep machines
Cable:
  bicep curl
  triceps pushdown
Curls
Dips: works triceps
Dumbbell:
  chest press: works triceps, shoulder
  overhead triceps press
Hammer curl: works biceps
Incline chest: works chest, triceps, shoulders
Kettle bell:
  one arm press
  push-up: works chest, back, arms, shoulders

push-down: works triceps
Push-up:
  knees: works chest, triceps, shoulders
  regular
  wall: works chest, triceps, shoulders
Rows
Shoulder press
Skull crusher: works triceps
Triceps kickback
Triceps machine
Triceps pull-down

Shoulders

Barbell:
  hang clean
Dips
Dumbbell:
  chest press: works triceps, shoulder
  front raise: works isolation
  lateral raise: works isolation
Front Raise (dumbbell, kettle bell, barbell, or resistance band)
Hang clean (dumbbell, kettle bell, or barbell): works shoulders, back
Incline chest: works chest, triceps, shoulders
Kettle bell:
  push-up: works chest, back, arms, shoulders
Lateral raise (dumbbell, kettle bell, or resistance band)
Push-up:
  knees: works chest, triceps, shoulders
  regular
  wall: works chest, triceps, shoulders
Rear deltoid raise
Rows
Shoulder press

Chest

Bench presses
Cable:
  chest press
  fly
Chest press machine exercises
Dumbbell:
  fly
Incline chest: works chest, triceps, shoulders
Kettle bell:
  push-up: works chest, back, arms, shoulders
Push-up:
  knees: works chest, triceps, shoulders
  regular
  wall: works chest, triceps, shoulders)

Abs

Abdominal crunches
Ab twist
Hanging leg raise
Kettle bell:
  power plank row
Plank

Back

Barbell:
  hang clean
  deadlift
Cable back row
Hang clean (dumbbell, kettle bell, or barbell): works shoulders, back
Kettle bell:
  push-up: works chest, back, arms, shoulders
  deadlift: works lower back, hamstrings
Lat pull-down
Rows
Superman: works lower back

Legs (hamstrings, quadriceps, calves)

Cable hamstring curl
Calf machines
Calf raise
Incline walking backwards
Kettle bell deadlift: works lower back, hamstrings)
Leg:
   curl: works hamstring isolation
   extension: works quad isolation
   press: works hamstring, quad)
Lunges
Side shuffles
Squats
Standing calf-raise
Step-ups
Thigh blaster: works quads)
Treadmill machine

Full Body

Burpee
Cardio exercises
Jumping Jacks
Kettle bell:
   swing
Power push press

Description of Exercises

Abdominal machines: Work abs, isolation lifts.

Abdominal crunch: Works abs.
- Bicycle
- Bosu ball
- Decline
- Exercise ball
- Medicine ball
- Oblique –as you tighten your abdominal muscles and lift up your head, twist to one side. Return to laying position. Repeat on other side.
- Physioball
- Regular
- Reverse
- Roman chair lift

Bicycle

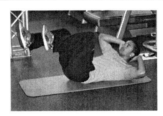 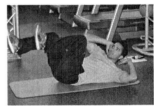

Bosu ball

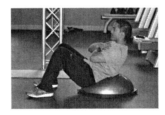 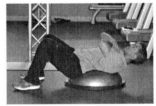

Decline

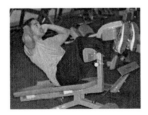 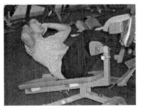 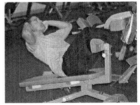

Exercise ball	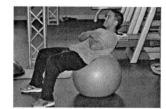	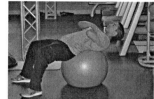
Medicine ball	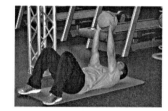	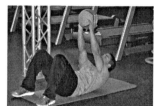
Physioball	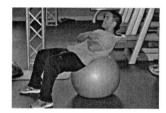	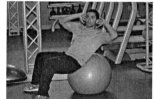
Regular abdominal crunch	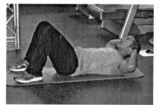	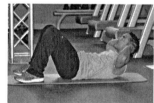
Reverse abdominal crunch	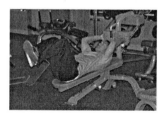	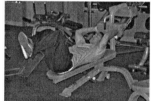
Roman chair lift	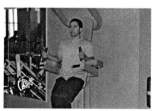	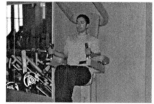

Ab twist: Works abs.

Remaining in a flexed position, with head off the floor (as you would be at the top of an ab crunch), rotate your abs and midsection from side to side keeping your abdominals flexed at all times.

Active recovery: (see *recovery*)

Alignment, general: (see also, *form*)

Core (abs) tight, natural alignment of spine (no arching back), toes facing forward (not pointing in or out), feet shoulder-width apart. Knees should never be hyperextended (locked tight) or bend further than lining up with your toes. Elbow should never extend to where arm is straight.

Arm circle: Works arms.

Arm circle

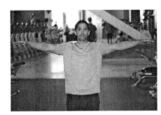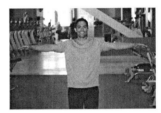

Back row seated: (see *row*)

Barbell:
- Bench press, works chest, compound lift
- Curl, works arms (bicep)
- Deadlift, works lower back, compound lift
- Hang clean, works shoulders and back
- Lunge legs, works legs (quads and hamstrings)
- Row, works back
- Squat, works legs (quads and hamstrings) (see also *squat*)

Bench press

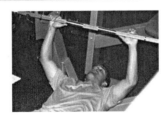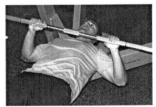

Curl

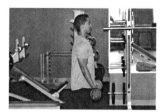 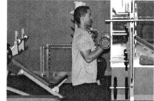

Deadlift

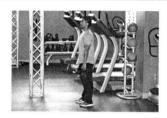 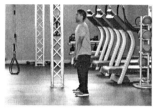

Hang
clean

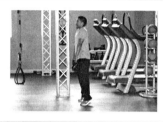 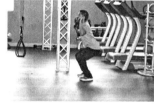

Lunge

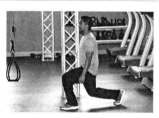 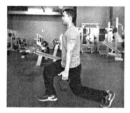

Row

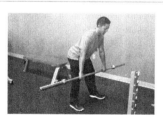 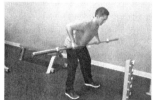

Squat

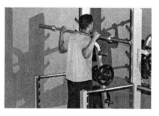 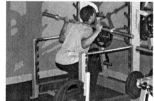

Bed dip: (see *dip*)

Bench, workout: A flat bench or adjustable bench that helps you to perform patters of resistance training.

Bench press: Works chest, compound lift.
- Barbell
- Dumbbell
- Dumbbell fly
- Incline
- Regular (if type of bench press is not described, the basic type of bench press is to use either the barbell or dumbbell)

Barbell

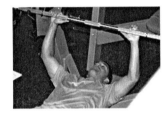 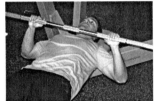

Dumbbell

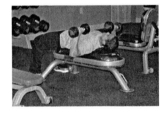 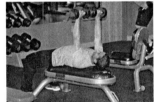

Dumbbell fly

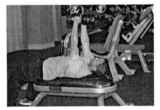 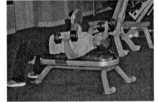

Incline

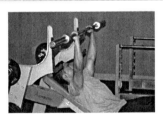 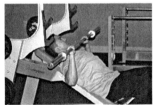

Bicep curl: (see *curl*)

Bicep machines: Works bicep, isolation.

Bicep machines

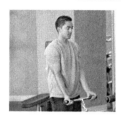 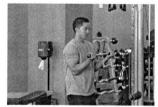

Bicycles: (see *abdominal crunch*)

Body weight squat: (see *squats*)

Bosu ball crunch: (see *abdominal crunch*)

Breathing: Exhale as the muscle contracts and inhale as the muscle releases with each repetition, and put 100 percent of your focus and energy on feeling your muscles contract and relax through every rep.

Burpee: Works full body. A push-up (see *push-up*) into a jump squat (see *squat*), all in one motion. Start in the push-up position, perform a push-up and then all in the same motion bring your body into a squat position and perform a jump squat.

Cable machine:
- Cable back row, works back
- Cable bicep curl, works arms (bicep), isolation
- Cable chest press, works chest
- Cable fly, works chest
- Cable hamstring curl, works legs (hamstring)
- Cable triceps pushdown, works arms (triceps)

Cable back row

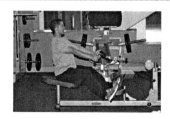 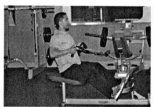

Cable bicep curl

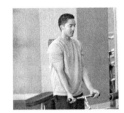 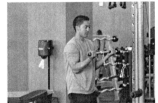

Cable chest press

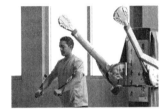 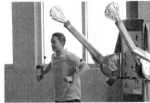

Cable fly

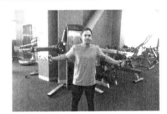 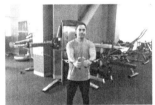

Cable hamstring curl

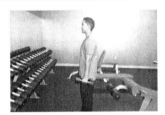 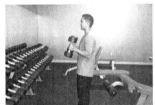

Cable tricep pushdown

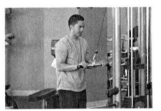 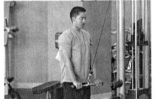

Calf machines

- Barbell calf raise
- Dumbbell calf raise
- Seated calf raise
- Standing calf raise machine
- Toe raises

Calf raise: Works legs (calf).

- Seated: While in a seated position with knees bent in a 90-degree angle (on a seated calf raise machine, or sitting on the edge of a chair or exercise ball with a weight on your knees), place your feet flat on the floor and slowly raise onto the balls of your feet, squeezing the calves as you go. For better range of motion, place a book or something under the balls of your feet, so you can drop your heels below as well as raise them above the level of your toes. Stay controlled and steady. Do not bounce.
- Standing: Start with a step and something to hold on to (the back of a workout machine or a chair). Place most of your weight on your toes, with heels hanging off the edge of the step. Drop the heels below the step, the raise up you're your toes so that your heel is above your toes. Repeat.

Cardio exercises:

- Elliptical
- Incline walking
- Interval training
- Jump rope
- Kickboxing
- Rowing
- Running
- Stationary bike
- Swimming
- Treadmill
- Training

  High-intensity training—using maximum effort separated by longer rest periods (similar to sprint training but longer rest periods).

  Incline walking—walking on an incline of 12 to 30 percent.

  Running uphill—running on an incline as part of either sprint training or sustained jogging or walking.

  Sprint training—running as fast as you can for short bursts followed by short rests.

Chair dip: (see *dip*)

Chest press machine: Works chest and shoulders.
- Hammer strength

Hammer strength

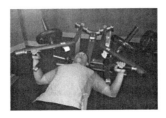 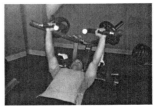

Compound lift: (see *lifts*)
Resistance exercises that focus on large muscle groups.

Crunch: (see *abdominal crunch*)

Curl: Works bicep, isolation lift.
- Barbell (see *barbell*)
- Dumbbell (see *dumbbell*)
- EZ
- Forearm/wrist
- Hammer
- Preacher

EZ

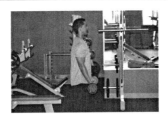 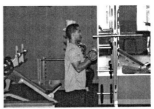

Forearm/wrist

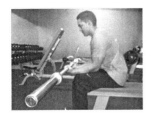 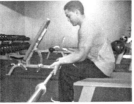 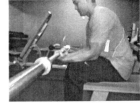

Hammer

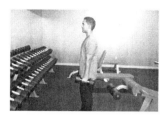 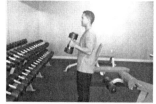

Preacher

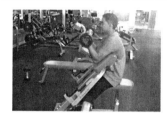 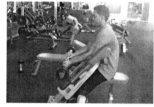

Deadlift: Works back.
Can be performed with a barbell, dumbbell, and kettle bell

Deadlift

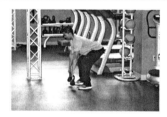 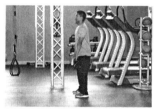

Dip: (also known as "bed dip" or "chair dip"), works shoulders and arms (triceps)

Dip

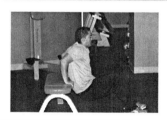 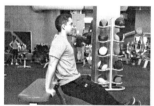

Dumbbell:
- Chest press, works chest, triceps, shoulder
- Curl, works bicep
- Fly, works chest
- Front raise, works shoulders, isolation lift
- Lateral raise, works shoulders, isolation lift
- Lunges, works legs (hamstrings and quadriceps)

- Overhead triceps press, works arms and shoulders
- Row, works back
- Squats, works legs (see *squat*)
- Triceps kickback, works arms (triceps) – create a tripod with your body by leaning forward with your left knee and left hand on a bench and your right leg straight on the ground. Your left arm should be positioned directly under your shoulder. Tighten your core. Hold the dumbbell with your right hand, and bring your upper arm back so it is in line or parallel with your back. Your elbow should be bent at a 90-degree angle. Keeping your elbow at your side, straighten your arm so that the forearm and hand holding the dumbbell move backward. Bend your elbow back to the 90-degree angle position. Keep the movement slow and controlled. Do not bounce. Repeat on opposite side.
- Walking lunges, works legs,

Chest press	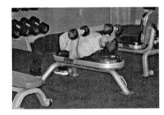	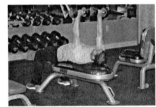
Curl	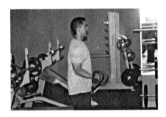	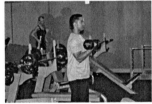
Fly	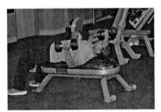	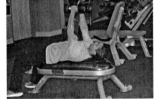
Front raise	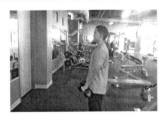	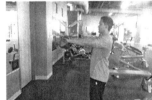

Lateral rise

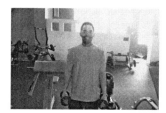 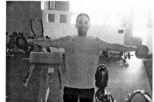

Lunges

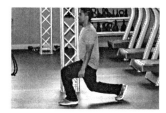 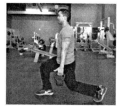

Overhead triceps

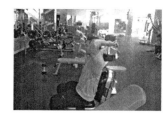 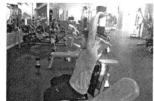

Row

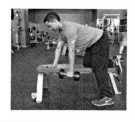 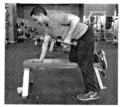

Triceps kickback

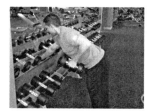 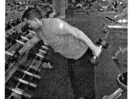

Walking lunges

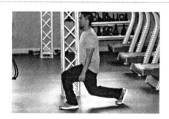 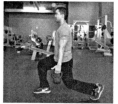

Effort: (see *intensity*)

Emphasize: (see *focus*)

Exhale/Inhale: (see *breathing*)

EZ bicep curl: (see *curl*)

FITT Principle: How to change up your workouts using frequency, intensity, time, and type.

> Frequency: Increase how many times per week or month you workouts.
> Intensity: Increase how hard you exercise by the speed of your cardio or how level of resistance during strength training.
> Time: Increase how long you do a single cardio exercise, and in resistance training, increase the number of sets per exercise, or move to more difficult types of lifts (see *Resistance Training*, chapter 5).
> Type: Change the activities and exercises in your workouts.

Focus: (Work during full-body workouts.) Doing a higher number of exercises using one muscle group or body area than another

Forearm/wrist curl: (see *curl*)

Form: Core (abs) tight, natural alignment of spine (no arching back), toes facing forward (not pointing in or out), feet shoulder-width apart. Knees should never be hyperextended (locked tight) or bend further than lining up with your toes. Elbow should never extend to where arm is straight.

Front raise: (see also *dumbbell*) Works shoulders, isolation lift. Can be performed with dumbbells, resistance bands, kettle bells, or barbell.

Front raise

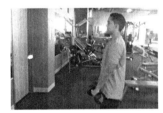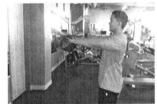

Full body:
- Resistance training guidelines
  (see *"Resistance Training,"* Chapter 5).

Hammer strength: (see *chest press machine*)

Hammer curl arms: Works biceps.

Hammer curl

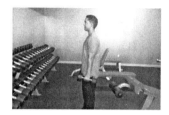 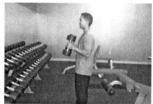

Hang Clean: Works shoulder and back.
Can be performed with kettle bells, dumbbells, or barbells.

Hang clean

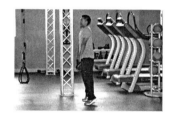 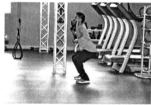

Hanging leg raise: Works abs.
Not for beginners. Using bars to hold your body off the ground, bring your knees up to your chest in a controlled fashion with very little momentum to help you.

Hyperextension

Hyperex-tension

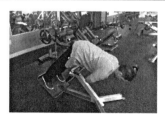 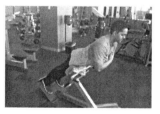

Hypertrophy: The building of lean muscle tissue.

Incline chest: Works chest, triceps, shoulders.

Can be performed using a machine, barbell, or dumbbell.

Incline
chest

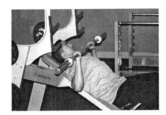 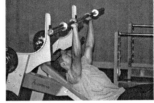

Incline bench press: (see *bench press*)

Incline walking backwards: Works legs (hamstrings, quads,

calf muscles). Walking backwards on a treadmill incorporates more quadriceps recruitment. Walk on the balls of your feet at a backwards incline, but be careful as you attempt to do this. Set the treadmill at a very slow pace until you get the feel for it. If you can't keep your balance on your toes, just try to keep your weight forward on your feet. Be sure that you are squatting down, leaning slightly forward to accomplish the most results. Stay in an athletic position. By sitting lower in your walk while going backwards, you strengthen your hamstrings as well.

Incline
walking
backwards

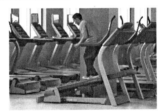 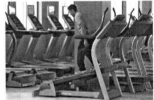

Inhale/Exhale: (see *breathing*)

Injury: (see also *sore muscles*) Feeling pain for an extended period of

time (a few days) or experiencing extreme pain during movement of any exercise. Check with your doctor.

Intensity: A level of effort. High intensity is to feel challenged. Low

intensity is to feel minimal effort. Intensity is *your* sense of how hard you are working.

Isolation exercises: An exercise that focuses on just one muscle.

Jump squat: (see *squat*)

Jumping jacks: Works full body.

Kettle bell:
• Deadlift: Works back and shoulders.

Deadlift

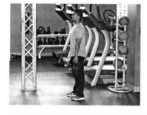 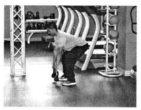 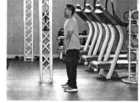

• One arm press: Works shoulders and arms. Begin with legs shoulder width apart, toes facing forward. With kettle bell at shoulder level, (if this is a right arm hold, palm should be facing left, and vice versa), elbow tucked in to ribs, and opposite arm straightened horizontally from shoulder for balance, push kettle bell straight up and straighten your elbow. Your palm will turn to face forward as you push the kettle bell up. You can give yourself momentum, by slightly bending your knees and inhaling just before you straighten your legs, exhaling, and pushing the kettle bell up to full extension of elbow.ok
• Power plank row: Works abs and back (see *power plank row*).
• Push-up: Works chest, back, arms, shoulders. A regular push-up except you place your hands on the handles of kettle bells rather than on the ground. It provides the opportunity for wider range of movement.
• Squat: Works legs. A regular squat (see *squat*), but while holding kettle bells.
• Swing: Works full body. Place feet a little wider than your hips and slightly bend your knees. Bend at hips a little less than 90 degrees, keeping back straight but crouching a bit. Holding a single kettle bell with both hands, start with kettle bell between and just behind legs, then with a quick thrust, straighten hips and raise arms until hands are about shoulder height (palms down). As you come up, tighten your glutes. Keep your neck inline with your back.

Lateral raise: Works shoulders.
Can be performed with dumbbell, kettle bell, or resistance band.

Lateral rise

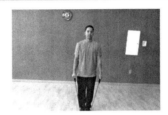 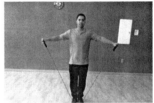

Lat pull-down: (see *pull-down*).

Leg
- Curl: works hamstring, isolation.
- Extension: works quadriceps, isolation.
- Pres: works hamstring and quadriceps.

Leg Curl

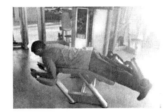 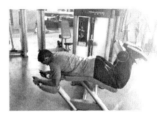

Leg Extension

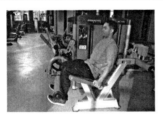 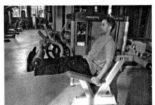

Lifts:
- Compound: Resistance exercises that focus on large muscle groups.
- Isolation: Resistance exercises that focus on a single muscle.

Lunge: Works legs.
Keep your body in an upright position with your core tight. As you lunge forward, make sure your knee lines up over your toes. Never go past your toes, in order to avoid injury.

- Regular/stationary: Start with feet together and hands on hips. Lunge one leg forward, then step back so feet are together again. Repeat with other leg.
- Treadmill: Slow the treadmill down to 1.5 miles per hour so that you can control the movement. The lunge on an incline (15 percent incline or higher; the higher the better) is the most effective exercise to do if you are trying to get deeper hamstring and gluteus recruitment. The incline lunge is a great exercise to incorporate as a super set (performing two exercises with no rest) with weight training for legs.
- Walking: Start with feet together and hands on hips. Lunge one leg forward, then put your weight on that same foot and lunge forward with the opposite leg in a forward moving pattern.

Mat, yoga, or rubber: Good for cushioning body during floor exercises and to protect floor if free weights are dropped on the ground.

Medicine ball crunch: (see *abdominal crunch*)

Military press: (see *shoulder press*)

Muscle groups, large:
- *Arms (biceps, triceps)*
- *Shoulders*
- *Chest*
- *Back*
- *Abs*
- *Legs (hamstrings, quadriceps, calves)*

Passive recovery: (see *recovery*)

Physioball crunch: (see *abdominal crunch*)

Plank: Works abs.

Plank

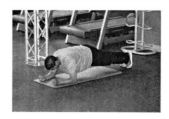

Plyometric exercises: Movement patterns done with bursts of energy such as jumping, jump squats, split squat jumps, and box jumps.

Position/posture: (see *form*)

Power push press: Works full body.
Bring kettle bells or dumbbells up to shoulders, with palms facing forward. Keep legs shoulder width apart with toes pointed forward. Do not move feet during this activity. Inhale for preparation. Then altogether: exhale, bend knees and in a continuous sweeping movement, using the momentum as you stand straight again, simultaneously push arms up over head, straightening elbows.

Power plank row: Works abs and back.
Start in a push-up position. Rather than having hands on the floor, place the kettle bells or dumbbells on the floor and hold the handles of the bells with your arms fully extended (elbows locked). Balancing your body weight on one arm (and both feet) while lifting bell upward to side of body. Return to original position and do opposite side.

Power plank row

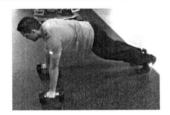 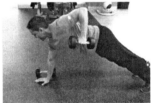

Preacher curl: (see *curl*).

Pull-down (also known as "lat pull-down"): Works back and arms.

Pull down

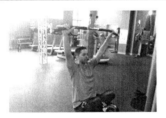 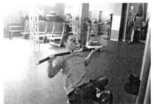

Pull-up: Works back, arms and shoulders. You can use overhand or underhand grip on the bar, at or slightly wider than shoulder width. Face forward (not looking up to bar) and pull yourself up so that the chin comes as close as you can (or above) the level of the bar.

Push-down: (see *triceps*)

Push-up:
- Knees: Works upper body, chest, triceps, shoulders.
- Regular: Works full body.
- Wall: Works upper body, chest, triceps, shoulders.

Push up: knee

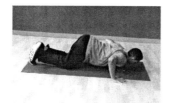 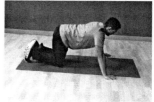

Push up: regular

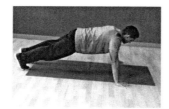 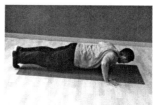

Push up: wall

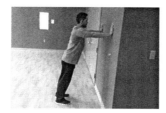 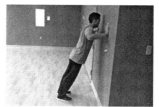

Recovery:
- Active recovery: Any low-intensity exercise (light cardio, low resistance).
- Passive recovery: Keeping the body at rest (or sleep)

Repetition (or, "rep"): the number of times you do an exercise without stopping. When using weights, repetitions should be controlled and take three to five seconds from start to finish of one rep (extension position to contraction and returning to extension position).

Rear deltoid raise: Works shoulders.

Keep core tight, feet hip-width apart. Hold dumbbellswith palms facing back. Keep your back and neck straight (head should not look up or down but stay in line with the spine) and lean forward from the hips to about an 80-degree angle (in other words, don't bend all the way down so that your back is parallel to the floor). Keeping your elbows straight, lift your arms out to the side (palms stay facing back). Keep your movements controlled.

Resistance band:

- Back row: Works back and arms (biceps).
- Bicep curl: Works arms (biceps).
- Shoulder lateral raise: Works shoulders.

Resistance back row

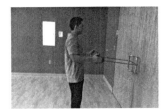 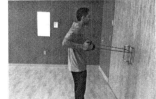

Resistance bicep curl

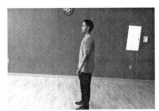 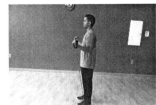

Resistance shoulder lateral raise

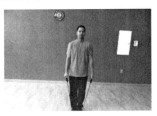 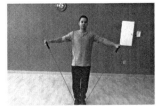

Resistance shoulder front raise

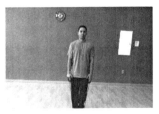 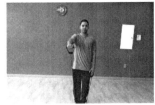

- Shoulder front raise
- Side shuffle: Works legs (hips).

  Start in athletic stance, with upper body bent slightly forward from the hip. Get on balls of feet and quickly bring feet closer together, then apart, moving sideways. It can help to have your hands held behind your back. This will keep your upper body aligned.
- Triceps extension: Works arms (triceps).

  Using a cable machine, or EZ curl bar, place feet together, slightly bend your knees, and keep core tight. Tuck your elbows in to your body and begin by holding the bar with your elbows slightly more than 90 degrees, then exhale while pulling down until elbows are straight.

Reverse crunch: Works abs (see *abdominal crunch*).

Roman chair lift: Works abs.

Roman chair lift

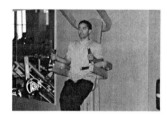 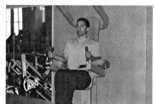

Rope triceps push-down: (see *triceps*)

Row:

- Barbell: (see *barbell*)
- Cable back row: (see *cable*)
- Kettle bell power plank row: (see *kettle bell*)
- Resistance band: (see *resistance band*)
- Seated back row, Works arms (bicep).
- Back row: Works back/deltoids.
- Upright back: Works arms and trapezius.

Row seated back

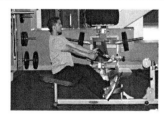 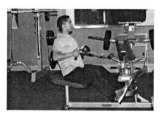

Row back row

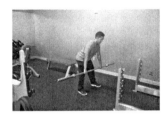 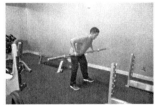

Row upright back

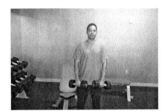 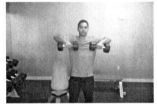

Set: A group of repetitions.

Shoulder press: (also known as *military press.*) Works shoulder and arms (triceps).

Shoulder press

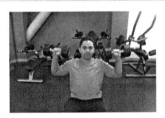 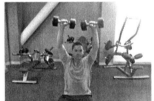

Side shuffles: Works legs.
Standing sideways on the treadmill, with your right leg toward the front end of the treadmill, take your first step with your right foot, then bring your left foot next to your right foot (almost touching) and then repeat. You should stay on the balls of your feet, keeping your core tight and controlling your body.

Sit-up: (also known as, see *abdominal crunch*)

Skull crusher: Works arms (triceps).

Skull crusher

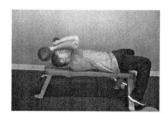 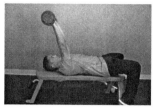

Sore muscles: The difference between sore muscles and an injury is that sore muscles can still move. They will feel tight, but not cause intense pain.

Split squat jump: The name is misleading, as there is no "squat" position in this jump. It is really a jumping lunge. Start in a lunge position, then jump into a lunge with the opposite leg, and repeat.

Squat: Works legs and gluteus.
Begin in a standing position with feet hip-width apart and toes pointing forward. Bend your knees to 90 degrees, until you are in a sitting position—(this is the "squat")—making sure knees never go past the point of your toes. With elbows straight, arms move straight in front of you from shoulder for balance. Don't arch your back. Return to standing position.
   • Barbell: barball held behind head on shoulders

Squat barbell

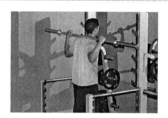 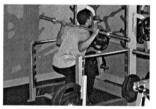

   • Body weight: This is a normal squat.
   • Dumbbell: A normal squat while holding dumbbells.
   • Jump: Start in a squat position, jump into the air and return to squat position. Repeat.
   • Kettle bell: A normal squat while holding kettle bells (see also *kettle bell*).

Standing calf-raise: (see *calf raise*)

Step-up: Works legs.
- Regular
- Side

Step up regular

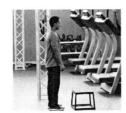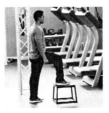

Step up side

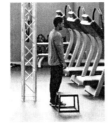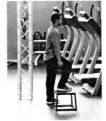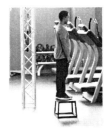

Stretch:
- Hamstring
- IT band
- Hamstring lower back
- Neck
- Quad
- Shoulder
- Upper back
- Groin stretch
- Calf stretch
- Chest stretch

Stretch hamstring

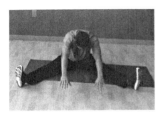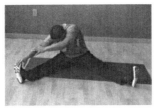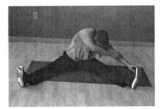

Stretch IT band

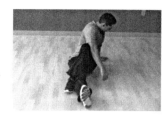 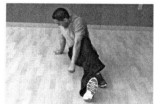

Stretch hamstring lower back

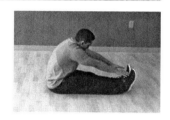

Stretch neck

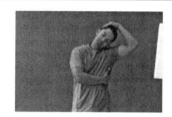

Stretch quad

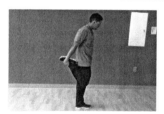 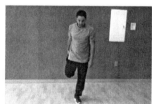

Stretch upper back

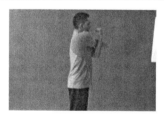 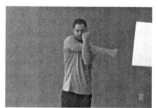

Stretch groin

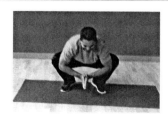

Stretch calf

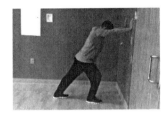 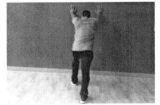

Stretch chest

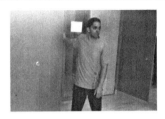

Superman: Works lower back.

Superman

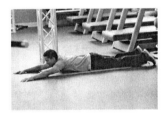 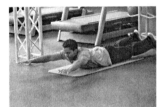

Thigh blaster: Works legs (quadriceps).

Thigh blaster

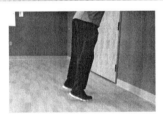 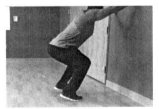

Treadmill: Works legs.

- Lunges: Works quadriceps, hamstrings.
- Side shuffles
- Walking backward incline: (on toes).

Treadmill, side shuffles

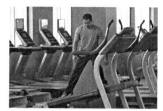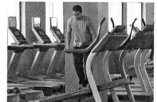

Treadmill, walking backwards

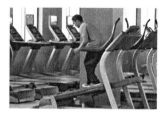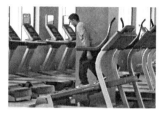

Triceps machines: Works arms (triceps), isolation.

Triceps: Isolations.
- Kickback: Holding a dumbbell, resistance band, or using a cable machine, keep your elbow level with your body and extend your arm to full extension, pointing the weight back.
- Push-down: Can be performed using cable machines, ropes, or EZ curl bar.

Triceps push down

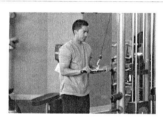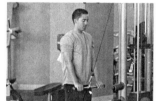

Walking lunge: (see *lunge*)

Workout programs: (see *"Putting it All Together,"* chapter 7)
Best balance is generally 20 minutes of cardio and 40 minutes of resistance training, depending on your goals. Workouts should increase in intensity but not time. Sixty minutes should be maximum workout time per day unless you are training for an athletic event.

Notes

Chapter 1: Getting Started

1. There are some adjustments to this general rule for beginners and those with specific body-shaping goals, which I'll discuss in each chapter.
2. "What is a healthy body fat percentage?" 2010. Online posting. National Academy of Sports Medicine. Commentary. Sharecare.com. June 2012.
3. Essential fat is the percentage of fat required for a woman or man to maintain her/his health.
4. National Heart, Lung and Blood Institute, National Institutes of Health. "Calculate Your Body Mass Index." Online. www.nhlbisupport.com. 28 Sept. 2012
5. The simplest means of taking your pulse is by using a heart rate monitor. It is something I recommend getting as you will use it daily to measure your progress. Otherwise, count your pulse for 15 seconds, then multiply that number by 4.

Chapter 2: The Missing Link: Mental Fitness

1. All clients' names have been changed for privacy.
2. Meyer, Paul J (2003) *Attitude is Everything: If You Want to Succeed Above and Beyond.* Meyer Resource Group, Inc. ISBN 978-0-89811-304-4.

Chapter 3: Nutrition Part I

1. Dolson, Laura. "List of High-Protein Foods and Amount of Protein in Each." 8 July 2009. Online. About.com. The New York Times Company. Aug. 2012.

2. Augustine, Jodi, RD CD. Clinical Review. "Carbohydrate Counting Examples." GroupHealth. 24 Feb. 2012. Online. www.ghc.org. Aug. 2012.

3. Boyers, Lindsay. "What Role Does Fat Have in Our Diets?" Reviewed/Updated by Shawn Candela 16 Jan. 2011. Online. Livestrong.com. Sept 2012.

4. USDA Center for Nutrition Policy and Promotion. "Dietary Guidelines for Americans, 2010." Released 31 Jan. 2011. Online. DietaryGuidelines.gov. July 2012.

5. Mayo Clinic. "Nutrition and Healthy Eating – Dietary Fats: Know Which Types to Choose." 15 Feb. 2011. Online. Mayoclinic.com. July 2012.

6. USDA Center for Nutrition Policy and Promotion. "Dietary Guidelines for Americans, 2010." Released 31 Jan. 2011. Online posting. DietaryGuidelines.gov. July 2012.

7. American Heart Association. "Know Your Fats." Updated 25 Jun. 2012. Online. 28 Aug. 2012.

Chapter 4: Nutrition Part II

1. All clients' names have been changed for privacy.

2. Chronic Dis. 2006 October; 3(4): A129. Published online 2006 September 15. www.ncbi.nlm.nih.gov/pmc/articles/PMC1784117

Chapter 5: Resistance Training

1. If you are focused on bulking up, you won't want to train every day as the muscles are being pushed to their maximum and need rest days. See "Bulking Up" sections in this and other chapters.

2. Reminder: Beginners should learn the fundamental movements before moving on to compound lifts that are a little more demanding on the body. The fundamentals to learn and practice include: keeping knees over toes on any lower body exercise, keeping back straight (never arch) when doing upper body exercises, and making sure that the body is aligned naturally. Again, you shouldn't ever feel an uncomfortable pinch while doing these exercises.

Chapter 6: Cardiovascular Fitness

1. Hillman, Charles H., Ph.D. et al. "Be Smart, Exercise Your Heart: Exercise Effects on Brain and Cognition." Jan 2008. *Nature Reviews Neuroscience*. Vol. 9, pp. 58-65.

2. Free Motion Fitness. "Exercise Benefits of Incline Training." 3 Mar 2008. Online. Freemotionfitness.com. May 2012.
3. See Exercise Glossary for definition of terms
4. FreeMotion Fitness. "Exercise Benefits of Incline Training: Applying Exercise Science to Enhance Training Effectiveness on the FreeMotion Fitness™ Incline Trainer." March 2008. Online. Freemotionfitness.com. I have been following many of FreeMotion Fitness' training recommendations for more than three years now and find it to be a very valuable program.

Chapter 7: Putting It Together

1. For a list of exercises to choose, see the "Build-Your-Own-Workout Menu" in this chapter and the "Exercise Glossary."
2. Twenty minutes is optimal if your goal is general fitness. If your goal is aerobic endurance you may want to increase that up to an hour of cardio.

About the Author

Greg Marshall has helped more than four thousand clients reach their fitness goals through his unique personal training programs. His experience includes large chain gyms and private programs. He publishes the daily fitness blog www.fiture.co and is published in the fitness professionals magazine *Club Industry*. He is currently the director of personal training at the gym at City Creek in Salt Lake City, Utah.

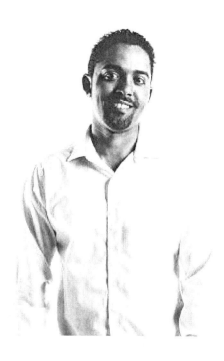

About the Publisher

Familius was founded in 2012 with the intent to align the founders' love of publishing and family with the digital publishing renaissance which occurred simultaneously with the Great Recession. The founders believe that the traditional family is the basic unit of society, and that a society is only as strong as the families that create it.

Familius' mission is to help families be happy. We invite you to participate with us in strengthening your family by being part of the Familius family. Go to www.familius.com to subscribe and receive information about our books, articles, and videos.

Website: www.familius.com
Facebook: www.facebook.com/paterfamilius
Twitter: @paterfamilius1 and @familiustalk
Pinterest: www.pinterest.com/familius

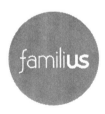

CPSIA information can be obtained at www.ICGtesting.com
Printed in the USA
BVOW040310150513

320715BV00005B/7/P